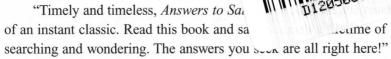

embark on 'real life'—or anyone else who wants to build a rich, rewarding, meaningful life!"

—**Kimberly Clark Sharp**, author of *After the Light*

"Jim Denney is a gifted writer and a gifted thinker. These *Answers* will not only satisfy you—they will get you to thinking and believing and doing."

—**Bert Decker**, author of *Speaking with Bold Assurance* and *You've Got to be Believed to Be Heard*

"Wisdom clothed in a lively, contemporary, conversational writing style. Full of thought-provoking concepts. I enjoy the way Jim Denney thinks as well as how he writes."

—**Muriel James**, coauthor of the classic *Born to Win: Transactional Analysis and Gestalt Exercises* (now in 22 languages) and author of *It's Never Too Late to be Happy*

"If you are on a quest for success, happiness, love, meaning, or God, this book is for you. Whatever you seek in life, *Answers to Satisfy the Soul* will speed you on your journey."

—**John C. Maxwell**, author of *The 21 Irrefutable Laws of Leadership* and *Be a People Person*; founder of The INJOY Group

---

"First, buy our new book. Then, if you have any money left over, buy *Answers to Satisfy the Soul*. (If you *still* have money left over, buy more of our books!) Jim Denney has more insight and practical wisdom than one human being should be allowed to have. Think of him as a sort of a cross between Norman Vincent Peale and Mark Twain—except Jim isn't dead yet. We especially liked that chapter on the meaning of life."

—**Bruce & Stan**, best-selling authors of *Bruce & Stan Search for the Meaning of Life*

"A thoughtful and passionate exploration of the many questions that puzzle modern folk, in a time of rapid change."

—**David Brin**, author of *The Transparent Society: Will Technology Force Us to Choose Between Freedom and Privacy?*, *Foundations Triumph*, and *Sundiver*

Answers to Satisfy the
SOUL

Answers to Satisfy the
SOUL

Clear, Straight Answers to 20
of Life's Most Perplexing Questions

Jim Denney

Clovis, California

Printed in the United States of America

Published by Quill Driver Books/Word Dancer Press, Inc.

8386 N. Madsen Avenue

Clovis, California 93611

559-322-5917 • 1-800-497-4904 • FAX 559-322-5967

QuillDriverBooks.com

Quill Driver Books titles may be purchased in quantity at special discounts for educational, fund-raising, business, or promotional use. Please contact Special Markets, Quill Driver Books/Word Dancer Press, Inc. at the above address or at 1-800-497-4909.

Quill Driver Books/Word Dancer Press, Inc. project cadre:
Doris Hall, John David Marion, Stephen Blake Mettee, Linda Kay Weber.

First Printing

To order another copy of this book, please call
1-800-497-4909

Visit Jim Denney at
WWW. Denneybooks.com

ISBN 1-884956-20-3

Library of Congress Cataloging-in-Publication Data

Denney, James D.
   Answers to satisfy the soul : clear, straight answers to 20 of life's most perplexing questions / by Jim Denney.
      p. cm.
   Includes bibliographical references
   ISBN 1-884956-20-3
      1. Spiritual life--Miscellanea. I. Title

BL624 .D3886 2001
100--dc21

2001031829

To my children
Bethany and Ryan

Two delightful souls
who always bring me great joy,
pride, and satisfaction

Contents

Introduction .... *xi*

Questioning Ourselves

1. Does Character Matter? *3*

2. How Do I Become Successful? *12*

3. How Can I Increase My Luck? *28*

4. How Can I Put More Time in My Day? *42*

5. How Do I Stop Worrying? *55*

Questioning Relationships

6. What is Love? *69*

7. How Can I Have a Better Relationship? *76*

8. How Can I Get Past Feeling Angry? *88*

9. Do I Have to Forgive Others? *99*

10. How Can I Forgive Myself? *107*

Questioning Life

11. How Can I Find Happiness? *119*

12. What Is Truth? *129*

13. What Is the Meaning of Life? *138*

14. Why is There Evil in the World? *151*

15. How Can I Get Past My Fear of Death? *170*

Questioning the Infinite

16. Does God Exist? *185*

17. What Is the Soul? *202*

18. Does Prayer Really Work? *224*

19. Do Miracles Really Happen? *233*

20. Is Religion Important? *252*

Notes *269*

In Appreciation... .... *274*

About the Author *276*

A Book That Surprised Even Me

This is not the book I intended to write.

Sure, I knew the *questions* from the outset—but the *answers* that emerged astonished me again and again. As I began my journey through these chapters, serendipity took over. Surprises multiplied. Synchronicities abounded. Some of the most satisfying answers in this book were discovered only *after* I began writing.

Standing at the foot of a three thousand-year-old sequoia profoundly affected my thinking about good and evil in the universe. A conversation with a near-death survivor revealed new insights into the qualia and qualities of the soul. Dialogues with Internet friends altered my thinking about scientific approaches to God. This book has been a bracing adventure for me; I hope it will be for you as well.

I've tried to write the kind of book I like to read—fun, informal, and user-friendly. I believe the insights in these pages are easy to understand and to apply to everyday life. Yet, far from being simplistic or superficial, these truths are profound and life-changing. They are the insights that have changed *my* life, and that's why I'm passing them along to you.

These twenty answers to life's most perplexing questions come from my own life experiences as man and boy, husband and father, reader and writer, and inquisitive observer of this amazing universe of ours. Many of these ideas come from conversations I've had with fascinating and accomplished people: successful CEOs, psychologists and psychiatrists, motivational speakers, scientists, philosophers, theologians, entertainers, authors, Super Bowl-winning football players, and even a supermodel. In these pages, I've distilled the best and most important insights I've discovered along the various highways, avenues, and detours I have taken in my soul's brief but interesting journey.

As I began the process of writing this book, I asked myself, "What are the most important questions people ask about life?" I drew up a list of over a hundred questions. They ranged from the practical to the philosophical, from "How can I cure insomnia?" (I wish I knew!) to "Is there life on other worlds?" (unanswerable—at least for now). Then I whittled that list down to the twenty questions in this book.

These twenty questions and twenty answers cover a spectrum of issues that are common to us all, from the everyday to the eternal, from the intimate to the infinite, from "How do I become successful?" to "What is love?" to "Does God exist?" These are the crucial questions we all strive to answer at one time or another.

I'm not so naive as to think that the answers that satisfy *my* soul will, in every case, satisfy *yours*. But woven into each of these chapters are suggestions, clues, and epiphanies that *just might* move you a little closer to finding your own answers.

My soul is well-satisfied with the answers I have discovered and now share in these pages. I wish you a satisfying soul-journey as well.

Questioning Ourselves

1

Does Character Matter?

$\mathbf{M}$r. Hess was a good husband, a loving father, and a devoutly religious Catholic. He was happily married, with five children who adored him. As a boy, he had been especially fond of animals and nature, so it was only natural that he took up farming as a young man. He prospered as a farmer for several years. Recognized for his administrative skills, he was offered a series of government posts, and he succeeded in each one.

Every morning, Mr. Hess would have breakfast with his family, then leave for work, often pausing in his well-tended garden to enjoy the colors and fragrances of the flowers. He would put in a long day at his job, conducting staff meetings, making important decisions, handling paperwork, issuing directives. At the end of each workday, his children greeted him at the front door. They were always happy to see him, because he was a tender and affectionate father—the kind you might remember from *Leave It To Beaver* or *Father Knows Best*. He often brought them little gifts. He spent a great deal of "quality time" with his children, playing with them or helping them with their homework.

It was a wonderful life for Mr. and Mrs. Hess and their children. He made good money, held a responsible position, and was highly respected. His loyalty, patriotism, and administrative skills had earned him the respect and trust of the nation's popular and beloved leader. That is why the leader of the nation—a man named Adolf Hitler—had rewarded Mr. Hess by placing him in charge of the expansion of the Auschwitz extermination complex in southern Poland. From the bedroom window of his secluded home in the country, Mr. Hess even could see the chimneys of the camp, sending up plumes of smoke from the crematoriums. There the bodies of those deemed "undesirable" by the Nazi state—primarily Jews, Poles, Gypsies, and homosexuals—were consumed by fire, day and night.

Rudolf Hess was raised to be obedient, to work hard, to live a productive life. He approached the operation of Auschwitz as if it were a large farm or factory. He was the architect of the plans that kept the assembly line of death moving efficiently. He met his quotas. He took pride in his work. He was extremely efficient. Over two million people died at Auschwitz during his administration of the camps.

Beloved family man. Devout Catholic. Mass exterminator. How did all of these roles come packaged within the mind and soul of a single human being? As Lyall Watson explains in *Dark Nature*, it was because Rudolf Hess had erected a mental wall of separation between his home life and his professional life, "living in one reality that was bestial and vile, and another that was nurturant and humane, commuting daily between the two for five productive years."[1]

In other words, Rudolf Hess was able to *compartmentalize* his life. He lacked *integrity*. Integrity is a character trait—the quality of being whole, undivided, and uncompartmentalized. Had there been integrity between Hess's professed religion, his love for his family, and his behavior toward mankind, he could never have ordered those two million deaths.

Is character important? Well, a few people of character and integrity in positions of power could have averted a Holocaust. So yes, in this instance at least, character, or the lack of it, was literally a matter of life and death.

But what about you and me? Does character matter in our everyday lives? Let's explore these questions for a moment.

What is character?

What do we mean by the word *character*? In the broadest sense, according to *The American Heritage Dictionary of the English Language*, character is simply "a distinguishing feature or attribute" of someone or something. In that sense, a person could be said to have "good" character attributes or "bad" character attributes. But the dictionary also defines character as "moral or ethical strength"—and that, I think, is what most people think of when they hear the word character.

For our purposes, let's define character as

> "the sum total of the ethical and moral traits you need to live a good and decent life."

In our increasingly secular society, there has been a trend away from an emphasis on ethics. And in our pluralistic society, it's simply impossible to get a broad-based consensus on the rules of morality, which descend primarily from religion.

But character, as we've defined it here, transcends morality and religion. Character transcends politics and philosophy. We may not all have the same views on what is proper sexual behavior. We may not worship alike. We may disagree on politics and philosophy. But the issue of character cuts across all those differences. An atheist can have as much character as a country parson. A Republican, Democrat, Libertarian, and Green may have different views but identical character traits. The "character issue" cannot be "owned" by any segment of the political spectrum, whether liberal or conservative or middle-of-the-road.

A person of character doesn't need a law to tell him not to cheat or steal. He knows that cheating or stealing would be a violation of his character. It would not just break a law, it would desecrate his soul. He could not lie and say, "I'm a person of character who happened to tell a lie." He would know that in the act of lying he had become a liar. A lie wouldn't just break a rule, it would stain his character.

The ancient Greeks had a high regard for character—much higher than we seem to have today. The Greek concept of character was embodied in the word *arete* (pronounced ahr-ay-TEE). The concept of *arete* was defined in the epics of Homer—the *Iliad* and the *Odyssey*—and there is no English word that conveys the full depth of that Greek word. *Arete* embraces our English concepts of virtue, honor, excellence, nobility, courage, prowess, self-control, duty, and loyalty. That is a lot of meaning for one little word—but that is how profound this matter of character is.

Character is the glue that holds an individual together. More than our views, attitudes, ideas, or beliefs, it is *character* that truly defines who and what we are as individuals—and as a society.

The qualities that make up character

Let's take a look at some of the qualities that make up this thing we call *character*.

First, the character quality of ***integrity***: As we have seen, integrity is the quality of being whole and uncompartmentalized. A person of integrity is exactly the same at home, at work, and at church or synagogue. He is the same person, behaving the same way, whether in public or in private, whether being watched by a crowd of thousands or totally alone and unobserved. Integrity holds all the other character traits together. If you have integrity, then you cannot be honest at home and a liar at the office—you will demonstrate consistent character in every phase of your life.

Next, the character quality of *honesty*. Question: Would you want your emergency appendectomy performed by a doctor who cheated his way through med school? Well, the Center for Academic Integrity in Nashville has recently sounded a wake-up call. After surveying 7,000 students on twenty-six college and university campuses from 1990 to 1995, the Center revealed that *nearly 80 percent* of students admitted to cheating at least once. Donald McCabe, associate provost at Rutgers University in Newark and founder of CAI, says we are witnessing a "dramatic increase" of cheating in the halls of academe—and he attributes the rise of dishonesty to poor adult role models and lack of character instruction by parents.[2]

Dishonesty has a real economic price tag. When someone shoplifts in a department store, the price of goods must be raised to cover what retailers politely call "shrinkage." When employees steal from the boss, prices must be raised again to cover the cost of dishonesty. The FBI estimates the loss to American businesses due to internal theft alone at between $40 billion and $200 billion a year.[3]

Gregory Slayton is one of the most phenomenally successful executives of the Internet-based "new economy." In January 1998, he took over a failing software company, MySoftware, Inc. Two years later, the stock of the company—now renamed ClickAction (NASDAQ listing: CLAC)—was trading *4,000 percent* above its January 1998 price. While I was working on this book, I had the pleasure of interviewing Gregory Slayton in his Palo Alto office. He told me one thing in particular that really stuck in my memory: "Character is more important in the new economy than ever before. Things move so quickly in e-business that there's often no time to get the lawyers involved in drawing up contracts. You have to operate on trust and a handshake. You have to know that the people you're dealing with are honest. If you can't trust each other, you can't do business."

Next, there's the character quality of *fairness*. People of good character are evenhanded and fair-minded. They live out the dream of Martin Luther King, Jr., who said in that powerful speech before the Lincoln

Memorial, "I have a dream that my four little children will one day live in a nation where they will not be judged by the color of their skin, but by the content of their character." His was a dream of fundamental human fairness. Fair-minded people treat everyone alike, regardless of such superficial distinctions as skin color, gender, religious conviction, sexual orientation, and so forth. You cannot be a person of character without being a person of fairness.

> "*A* person of character doesn't need a law to tell him not to cheat or steal. He knows that cheating or stealing would be a violation of his character."

The character quality of *compassion* is also essential to good character and to a healthy society. Few Americans knew very much about Jordan's late King Hussein. But the Jordanian people knew him well and grieved deeply when he died of cancer in early 1999. Why? In large part, because he was a man of compassion. A young woman named Zwein Madi was a beneficiary of the king's kindness. When a friend of her family asked King Hussein to help with the treatment for Zwein Madi's rare and painful genetic disorder, the king didn't hesitate. He took care of all the bills—more than $20,000—out of his own pocket.

The king regularly listened to a morning call-in show on Jordan Radio. People sometimes called in with needs, problems, and crises, many involving children. He often picked up the phone, called the radio station, and solved the caller's problem on the spot. For example, when a bus driver, a father of eight, asked for help getting a heart operation for his seven-year-old daughter, King Hussein not only paid for the $5,000 operation, but thousands more in postoperative treatments.

And, King Hussein did not just practice "checkbook compassion." When a military pilot was severely burned in a helicopter crash, the king visited the pilot almost daily throughout his treatment and recovery. There were many people whose medical cases he followed personally, making calls and personal visits, talking to doctors, and following up. There are literally hundreds of stories of the compassionate acts of Jordan's King Hussein. He didn't do these compassionate deeds for "good PR" or political advantage—after all, you don't elect kings. He did them for the same reason he gave his people paved roads, modern irrigation systems, and improved agricultural technology: He truly cared about his people.

When King Hussein's successor, his son Abdullah, ascended to the throne, there were many doubts and questions: Would King Abdullah be strong enough to fill the political vacuum created by King Hussein's death? Equally important, would Abdullah be compassionate like his father? The doubts about the U.S.-educated Abdullah were intensified by his eccentric tastes for American blue jeans, *Star Trek* memorabilia, and Tex-Mex food.

But King Abdullah quickly silenced his critics with his strong leadership. Most important, King Abdullah not only continued the tradition of his father's compassion, but took it a step further. Several times since becoming Jordan's new king, he has disguised himself as a taxi driver or common laborer, going out among his people to find out how they live, what they think, and what they really need from his government. For example, he spent a day in disguise in a government hospital in Zarqa, observing how doctors treated (and mistreated) patients. His visit resulted in major reforms at that hospital and other government hospitals around Jordan. As a result, the people have embraced the new king as a worthy successor to his compassionate father.[4]

Generosity—the spirit of altruistic giving—is another essential Quality of character. Philosophy professor Loren Lomasky of Bowling Green State University recalls the time he was seated by his friend, an economist, aboard a plane preparing to take off. The plane was nearly full when a young family came down the aisle—a dad, a mom, and a babe-in-arms. Because they had boarded late, they couldn't be seated together. The father was put in a middle seat, many rows behind his wife and child. But shortly before takeoff, the passenger on the aisle next to the father offered to trade seats with the mother and her baby.

"Looks to me like market failure," said Lomasky to the economist. "That fellow gave up the better seat without compensation. Don't you think it would be more efficient to have a market in passenger seat rights?" In reply, the economist suggested that the passenger traded seats (a) in order to avoid guilt feelings, or (b) to obtain selfish pleasure from doing a good deed.

"This was explanation enough for my friend," Lomasky concluded. "Subsequently, we chatted about design possibilities for airplane-seat auctions and the failings of the Republicans." But sometime later, another possibility occurred to Lomasky: Perhaps, he pondered, "the passenger acted out of generosity."[5] Ah, generosity! Sheer human altruism! What a quaint idea! Could it be that a person could actually have the trait of generosity built into his character? And wouldn't the world be a better place if it were filled with people of generosity!

And then there is *tolerance*—what a much-needed character trait *that* is in these times! But what exactly *is* tolerance? Simply put, to tolerate is to put up with something, even if you don't agree with it or like it. True tolerance is a "live and let live" attitude. A tolerant person is able to say, "I don't have to agree with other people or like what they say or do, but if they're not harming anyone, let them be."

Some people like to say, "I'm tolerant of everything but intolerance." I suggest those people learn to tolerate a little intolerance. Some people have seemingly "intolerant" attitudes about certain things, and often those attitudes come from their religion, from the scriptures that they consider sacred. Should you and I tell them they have no right to believe what their religion teaches? If we don't tolerate their "intolerance," what have we become? Antireligious bigots! We have become intolerant of another person's religion! My friend Conor Northup shared a brilliant *reductio ad absurdum* with me, penned by Canadian journalist Ted Byfield:

> To believe anything at all is to believe it true. To believe something true is to believe that whatever is incompatible with it must be false. And to believe somebody else's belief false is implicitly intolerant. Therefore, if intolerance is an evil, belief itself—in anything—is an evil. So the only way we can get rid of intolerance is to prohibit belief. Which, of course, would be very intolerant indeed.

So let's build the character quality of tolerance into our own lives, and let's learn to even tolerate what may seem a bit intolerant to our "enlightened" selves. Even if we don't like what some people do, say, or think, as long as it doesn't hurt anyone, let's put up with it.

So many character traits, so little time. There's *self-control*—the ability to master one's behavior and impulses. There's *diligence*, often called a "work ethic," the character trait of a person who strives for excellence, who is never satisfied with "good enough," and is ambitiously dedicated to reaching his or her highest potential. There's *patience*, the quality of being able to defer immediate gratification in favor of a better reward down the road.

There's **perseverance**, determination, persistence, unstoppability, or what Walt Disney used to call "stick-to-it-ivity." There's **courage**, the willingness to take risks, face obstacles, withstand opposition, and brave dangers in the defense of a worthwhile cause or the pursuit of a worthwhile goal. There's **rationality**, the commitment to sound reasoning as a path to understanding and a guide to behavior. There is **self-reliance**, the ability to take responsibility for one's own life and actions; a self-reliant person has confidence in his or her own ability to make independent decisions and does not shift blame for mistakes onto others.

You may have some character qualities in mind that I didn't list. In these few pages, I have tried to be thorough, but I don't pretend to be exhaustive. The point is this: Yes, character matters. It matters to each of us as individuals. It matters to relationships. It matters to society. Without people of character, society could not exist.

Character and decision-making

How, then, do we build good character? Answer: *by making good choices*. Character is a by-product of the choices we make on a consistent, daily basis. Here are some choices that lead to good character:

Stop living to impress others. Don't fake it; be real. Make sure you are the same person in private that you are in public. Make a daily commitment to say what you mean and mean what you say. Choose to accept full responsibility for your mistakes, offenses, and flaws—without evasions, excuses, or blaming others. Choose to deal fairly and compassionately with everyone you meet. When confronted with a tough decision, ask yourself, "What is the courageous thing to do in this situation?" Commit yourself to doing what is difficult and right instead of what is easy and cowardly. Choose to accept challenges, because mastering challenges builds character.

Life is about making choices. I often hear people say, "I have a decision to make, and I'm confused about what I should do." That is rarely true. Usually, there is no confusion whatsoever about what a person *should* do. The confusion is between what he *wants* to do and what he knows is the *right* thing to do. For people of character, these decisions are fairly simple—they do the difficult but right thing, and they suffer few regrets.

Maybe you've had a friend who said something like this to you: "I'm torn between being faithful to my wife and having a fling with a woman at the office." For a person of weak character, this is a major dilemma. But for a person who has character qualities of integrity, honesty, and self-control? Hey, that's a no-brainer.

The person of little character always has an excuse. "Be faithful to my wife?" he says. "When this sweet young thing at the office is coming on to me every day? Easier said than done!"

Look, *everything* is easier said than done. Going to work every morning is easier said than done. Brushing your teeth is easier said than done. A person of character accepts reality and does what needs to be done.

> "*Choose to accept challenges, because mastering challenges builds character.*"

People of character don't whine, "I can't choose! If I become an astronaut, I can't become a supermodel! If I buy the Lexus, I can't have the Mercedes! If I order pizza, I can't have Szechwan! If I marry Jerry, I can't have Joey! If I choose one, I'll lose the other!" Every choice entails a loss. If you take the road that forks right, you can't go left. Nobody gets to have it all. Everybody makes choices.

Some would say, "But that's too tough!" Of course, it's tough. Everything worth doing is tough. Interviewing for a job is tough. Running a marathon is tough. Getting a degree is tough. Losing weight is tough. Quitting cigarettes is tough. Getting off drugs or booze is tough. Maintaining a healthy relationship is tough. Resisting temptation is tough. Raising kids is tough. Writing a book is tough. Life itself is tough— really, really tough.

It takes a lot of moral, ethical strength to live a good and decent life. It takes all the integrity, compassion, self-control, perseverance, and courage we can muster. It takes all of that—and more.

And that's why character matters.

2

How Do I Become Successful?

I love my job.

Over the years, my work as a writer has brought me into contact with an eclectic assortment of fascinating, *successful* people—from Supermodel Kim Alexis to Super Bowl champions Reggie White and Bob Griese to some of the top superexecutives in the country. I've questioned them, worked with them, and watched them in their public and private moments. I've gotten to know some of them very well.

And I've figured it out! I *know* where success comes from.

Living a successful life is not a matter of "hitting life's lottery" or being "born lucky." The common denominator in the lives of all the successful people I've known is the *decisions* they make about the way they live their lives. Here is what I have discovered—the Seven Undeniable Rules for a Successful Life.

1. Define what success means to you.

I first met Kim Alexis at her home in Laguna Hills, California. It was a beautiful home, but not pretentious—a warm and friendly family haven, not a palatial estate. The front yard was happily littered with toys— a tricycle, a kid-size basketball hoop, rubber balls, and the like—the unmistakable evidence that three active, happy boys lived there. Kim met me at the door, all smiles and warm California hospitality. She wore blue jeans, her hair was up in a ponytail, and she wore little makeup. I felt distinctly overdressed in my suit and tie, but Kim quickly put me at ease, beginning with a quick tour of her home.

In the living room, there was a stunning painting of Kim, a gift from an artist friend. The walls were hung with framed hockey and basketball jerseys (including a Bulls jersey signed by Michael Jordan), some of Kim's magazine photos, and other memorabilia. There was even a framed copy of the script for the final episode of *Cheers* (in which Kim guest-starred), signed by the entire cast. You remember that show. Whenever her name was mentioned by Sam or Norm or Cliff the Mailman, it was never just "Kim Alexis"—it was always "stunning Supermodel Kim Alexis" or "electrifying Supermodel Kim Alexis" or "dazzling Supermodel Kim Alexis."

But the Kim Alexis who invited me into her home that day was just Kim from upstate New York, your average girl next door (who just happens to be a supermodel). She took me out onto the deck behind her home, an enclosed grassy area backed by a steep hill. A few sheep and goats lay together under a tree at one end of the yard, shading themselves from the July sun.

Back inside, Kim introduced me to her husband, Ron Duguay, and then we sat down to talk. Though I was there to interview her, it wasn't like a business meeting at all. I soon put my clipboard of prepared questions away, and we just chatted about life and work and values and whatever came to mind. As I do with most people I interview, I put this question to Kim: "What does 'success' mean to you?" I thought I knew how she would answer. She's the most photographed model ever, with over five hundred magazine covers to her credit; she's appeared in theatrical films and TV movies and was the fashion editor of ABC's *Good Morning America* for several years; she has lived the fast-lane, Studio 54 lifestyle, with all the money and celebrity power that goes with it.

But when I asked her that question, her answer had nothing to do with what most people think of as success. She said, "To me, being successful means that Ron and the kids and I are together as a family, loving each other and collecting memories. The most important thing to me is that we are successful as a family."

"What about money, fame, and career?" I asked.

"That's important, of course," she said, "but my life doesn't revolve around money and career. It's about spending time with Ron and my kids. That's where true meaning and satisfaction in life are found. Ron and I live near L.A., and we could do the celebrity scene every night of the week. That kind of lifestyle spells 'success' to a lot of people, but that's not where our values are."

I heard a strikingly similar definition of success when I went to

Knoxville, Tennessee, to spend three days with the "Minister of Defense" of the Green Bay Packers, Reggie White. That was in the spring of 1996, about nine months before Reggie collected his first championship ring in Super Bowl XXXI. We talked about the fact that, while he was already a living NFL legend, assured of a place in the Hall of Fame, he had never won a championship at any level in his life—not in high school, nor in his college career, nor in his professional career. So I asked him, "If you finished your career without a championship, would you still consider yourself a success?"

"Jim," he said, "no matter what happens, I've got my stats and my place in the Hall of Fame, and nobody can ever take that away. But none of that stuff means success to me. My goals in life are to be the kind of man God wants me to be, to be a good husband to my wife Sara, and to be a good father to my children. If I've done all that, then I'm a successful man."

So the first step in achieving success is to define what success means to you, to have a clear picture in your mind of what success looks like. If success, to you, is defined as "the lifestyles of the rich and famous," fine, go for it. But I've known a number of people who were successful by that measure alone—and they were completely miserable. To me, a rich, famous, celebrated person who has no satisfaction in life is a failure, not a success.

Are wealth and status unimportant then? Not at all. But material success shouldn't be the *only* measure of success—and for some people, material success won't even enter into the equation at all. It is possible to be spectacularly successful in life even if you don't have two dimes to rub together. Here are a few examples:

- Saint Francis of Assisi gave up a huge inheritance to pursue a lifetime of faith and helping others. He took a vow of poverty—yet he was an enormous success.

- Cesar Chavez never earned more than $6,000 a year. His goal, however, was not personal wealth, but justice for American farm workers. Today, Chavez is a hero to many, and California remembers his birthday with a statewide holiday.

- Wangari Maathai, the founder of Kenya's Greenbelt Movement, does not live the lifestyle of the rich and famous. In fact, she has endured beatings, harassment, and vicious character assassination. But Wangari Maathai has been incredibly successful in reforesting Africa, defending the global environment, and championing the rights of women around the world.

So how do *you* define success? There's no right or wrong answer—but you can't ignore the question. You must know what you are aiming for in life. If you don't know what success is supposed to look like, how will you recognize it when you get there?

2. Dream big dreams.

Near the end of my three days working with Reggie White, he told me he wanted to make a bold prediction in his autobiography. "We're going to the Super Bowl this January," he said, "and we're gonna win it."

"You want to make that prediction in print?" I said. "That book will come out in September, and it will still be on the shelves in January. Aren't you worried that you'll look a little foolish if Super Bowl XXXI comes around and the Packers aren't in it?"

"Let me tell you something," said Reggie. "This past season ended for us when we lost the NFC title game in Dallas. After that game, we got on the team bus, and we were mad. Nobody was saying nothing. And Brett"—that's Brett Favre, the Packers quarterback—"came over to where I was sitting. He was crying and he took me by the shoulders and he said, 'Big Dog, I promise you, we're gonna win it all next season. We're going to the Super Bowl, and we won't let nothing stop us this time.' I said, 'I know we are.' So we *are* going to the Super Bowl, and we *are* gonna win it. That's a promise we're gonna keep."

So Reggie's autobiography, *In the Trenches*, came out in September of 1996, and Reggie's promise of a Super Bowl win appeared on the second from the last page of that book. When Brett Favre and Reggie got to training camp, they both began pumping up their teammates about going all the way. Favre even bragged to reporters, "We're gonna win the Super Bowl. Don't believe me? Then bet against me. I'm telling you right now: This year, it's Super Bowl or bust."

That season, the Packers played an incredibly tough schedule—no teams with a less than .500 record. They lost one player after another to injuries, yet they battled against adversity, stayed focused, and finished the season 13 and 3, tacked on two more wins in the playoffs, then defeated New England in the Super Bowl, 35 to 21. As I watched the game at home with my family and saw Reggie taking his victory lap around the Louisiana Superdome with the Lombardi Trophy held high above his head, I couldn't help thinking about that prediction he had made to me some nine months earlier: "We *are* going to the Super Bowl, and we *are* gonna win it."

Reggie's boldness in making that prediction *in print* made a powerful impression on me. I learned something important that year: Successful people set big goals in order to achieve great things. We are all capable of much more than we can imagine—so why not imagine the ultimate?

3. Focus on your dreams.

Everybody dreams of success. Only a few ever reach it. Why? Because success demands that we remain intensely, relentlessly focused on our dreams. Only a rare few have the level of focus it takes to keep faith with their dreams and see them through to triumphant completion. A dream only becomes reality if you stick to it.

The world is full of people who dream of writing that novel or building that dream house or starting a business. "Sure, I could do that," they say, "and someday I just might." But they never do and they never will. They keep their dreams in a shoebox, tied up with string, shoved under the bed—because they lack the courage to put their dreams to the test.

I remember when I first decided to take the plunge into fulltime freelance writing—no more paychecks every two weeks, no retirement plan, no paid vacation. I talked to a couple of writers who had been in the business for ten years or more. One told me, "You happened to call just as I'm quitting freelancing and taking a job with a publishing house. Jim, I just couldn't take it anymore. My advice is: Don't even *think* of freelancing unless you have at least a year's worth of living expenses saved up." Well, to do that I'd have had to rob a bank!

The other writer I talked to had over five million copies of his various books in print—and he did all his writing in his spare time. From 9 to 5, he headed up a nonprofit organization. He told me, "Don't quit your day job. Do your writing on evenings and weekends, and make sure you have a regular paycheck." Not much encouragement there, either.

I had a house (with a mortgage) to lose, plus a wife and two small children. And I had my dream of being a writer. What should I do? Should I listen to those veteran writers who advised me (with complete justification) not to even consider such a foolish move? Or should I pursue my dream? I went for the dream. And it was *tough*—incredibly tough.

But today, earning decent advances and royalties, I consider myself successful, and I know that more success is on the way. But the key to success in writing or any other endeavor is *focus*. You have to focus on the work at hand, regardless of distractions and interruptions. You have to focus on moving forward, no matter what obstacles are in your way. You have to focus on your goals, despite rejection and setbacks.

Richard Hooker spent seven years writing his Korean War comedy novel *M*A*S*H*. He submitted it to twenty-one different publishers before William Morrow & Co. finally published it. The book became an immediate best-seller and spun off a hugely successful movie and TV series—but it wouldn't have happened without Hooker's intense focus.

Lisa Alther wrote for twelve years and collected 250 rejection slips before making her first fiction sale. That first book, *Kinflicks*, was praised by critics who compared Alther to Mark Twain and J.D. Salinger. *Kinflicks* and Alther's later books, such as *Original Sins* and *Other Women*, have been enormously successful—but it never would have happened if she hadn't stayed focused during those twelve lean years of rejection.

Mystery writer Donald Westlake used to paper the walls of his apartment with rejection slips. The day he sold his first story to a magazine, he celebrated by ripping those rejection slips off the wall—all 204 of them! Today, with over seventy novels to his credit, he is one of the most successful writers in America—but he never would have gotten anywhere without a laserlike focus on his dreams.

An aspiring young cartoonist was told his drawings were not good enough for his high school yearbook. He applied to Disney and was turned down. His "Li'l Folks" comic strip was rejected by every major newspaper syndicate—but Charles Schulz persisted until, in 1950, he sold it to United Features Syndicate, which renamed it "Peanuts." Ultimately, "Peanuts" was carried daily by 2,600 newspapers in seventy-five countries, generating $1 billion a year in merchandising and spin-off revenue. Charles Schulz focused on his dreams and made Charlie Brown a household name.

So you want to be a success? Simple! All you have to do is *focus on your dreams*. For how long? *However long it takes.*

4. Be the best you can be.

To be a success, be the best. Not one of the best. Not second best. *The best.* If you're not striving to be the best, why bother? Why attempt anything if you're not going to give it your all?

Permit me another Reggie White story: Reggie is the best at what he does—and I know why. Reggie *works* at being the best. He's fanatical about staying in condition, even in the off-season. He is obsessed with excellence, as his NFL career record of 199 sacks—more than any other player in football history—clearly attests.

When I was in Knoxville, he took me to the private training room behind his home. You go past the Olympic-size indoor pool, through the double glass doors, and you're there: a sunny, spacious workout room with a huge TV set and stereo system, a Reggie White-trademarked weight machine, Reggie White exercycle, Reggie White treadmill, and a heavy-duty top-of-the-line Stairmaster. He put on the CD *So Much 2 Say* by Take 6, jumped onto the Stairmaster, set it to max resistance, and put himself through an inhumanly grueling workout. As he pumped and strained on that machine, I could feel the awesome might and energy of six-foot-five-inch, two hundred ninety-five-pound Reggie White vibrating the floor beneath my feet. I only know of two people in the world who could go through a workout like the one I saw—and the other one wears a cape and a red S on his chest.

Understand, this was in the springtime. Training camp and football season were still weeks away—yet Reggie worked out every day as if the game of his career were just around the corner. Whereas a lot of NFL players goof around in the off-season and report to training camp with a potbelly and a lot of bad habits, Reggie worked hard, day-in, day-out, to keep himself in fighting trim all year 'round. No one had to tell him to work hard. He worked hard because he was committed to being the best.

Watching Reggie work out, I knew I was in the presence of the most powerful human being I had ever met. I have been privileged in recent years to see some absolutely amazing feats, from the backboard-shuddering stuffs of Shaquille O'Neal to the graceful aerobatics of Michael Jordan. But for sheer, awe-inspiring physical might, I have never, ever seen the likes of the Minister of Defense.

After Reggie finished his workout, we sat on the sofa in his weight room and talked for an hour or so about his years with the Philadelphia

Eagles and the Green Bay Packers. Then he showered and we went back into the house for a lunch of Hardee's fried chicken. We sat at the kitchen table and I had a chicken thigh and some barbecue beans and cole slaw, while Reggie proceeded to demolish the better part of an entire chicken—he must have had five or six pieces piled on his plate at once. He tilted the bucket toward me and said, "Is that all you're having? Take another piece."

"No, thanks," I said. "I've got plenty."

"Aw, c'mon!" he said, grinning, "you've gotta have some more! You're gonna make me look bad!"

As if there was any way *I* could make *him* look bad! If I could go half an hour on the Stairmaster at full resistance, maybe I could get away with eating half a bucket of fried chicken, too—but I'm just a sedentary writer-type. When a person works as hard as Reggie to stay in condition, you know that every last ounce of that fried chicken is going to be converted into bone-crunching, quarterback-flattening muscle.

Millions of people have seen Reggie White, the finished product, bullrushing the offensive line, leaping clear over the top of a cut-blocking tackle, and gobbling up quarterbacks like so much Hardee's chicken. But I've seen something most people don't get to see: I've seen the product *being built*. I've seen the sweating, straining, hard-working Reggie White, committed to excellence, committed to being the best.

There's no shortcut to success. No matter what your goal, hard work is the key to getting there.

5. Stay loose and have fun.

Another football story. I met with Super Bowl champion Bob Griese and his son Brian just a few months after Brian won the Rose Bowl as quarterback of the undefeated Michigan Wolverines. We sat in the study of Bob's beautiful golf villa in the Blue Ridge Mountains of North Carolina. As we talked, Bob and Brian told me about the father-son discussion they had in a Pasadena restaurant, just a few days before the Rose Bowl.

"Brian," Bob had told his son, "there's no pressure on you. You've gotten to where you want to be. Now just go out there and have fun!"

Brian laughed. "I'm gonna have fun, Pops," he replied, "but I'm also gonna win the Rose Bowl!"

"I wanted Brian to stay loose," Bob explained. "I didn't want him feeling a lot of extra pressure just because it was a big bowl game. I told him to approach the Rose Bowl like any other game of the season—if he did that, I knew he'd be okay. I said, 'The Rose Bowl is just a football field like any other. It's a hundred yards long and fifty yards wide. You don't have to throw the ball any different than you've been throwing all year.'"

Well, that's the way Brian approached the big game. He stayed loose. He had fun. And despite throwing an early interception, despite falling behind early in the game, despite having to battle his way through a very tough, close game, Brian led his fellow Wolverines to a 21 to 16 victory over Washington State—and to Michigan's first national title in fifty years. Since then, Brian has gone on to succeed the fabled John Elway as starting quarterback of the Denver Broncos.

Brian always seems to have the *most* fun when things are tough, when there is adversity. "Sometimes I set up to throw," Brian told me, "and all of a sudden this big lineman's paw comes outta nowhere and rakes across my face mask. Right then, the pressure is intense and I have to make some crucial decisions. The pocket is collapsing, and the defensive line is charging—but that's what makes it *fun*.

"One time we were losing to Ohio State and I was subbed in after our starting quarterback was hurt. I knew the Ohio State defense was tough, but kind of overanxious, you know? They were thinking, *Griese is just a backup quarterback. We'll chew him up and spit him out.* I mean, they would have just loved to get in there and bury me. So I thought, *Fine, let's have some fun with this.*

"Anytime a defensive lineman or a linebacker blitzes, he comes at you so fast that any little move you make, man, he's going to fly right past you. It makes them look terrible—and it's funny! I'd say to them, 'Hey, you've got to learn to lay back, man, because you'll never get me that way.' And they'd say, 'I'll get you next time, Griese! Next time I'm coming from your back side!' But they didn't get me. I just kept having fun with them, and by the end of the game, we'd won.

"There was another game that season, against Iowa in Michigan Stadium, and I really struggled in the first half. I threw three interceptions, and Iowa got two touchdowns off those interceptions. At halftime, we were down 21 to 7. When we came out to play the second half, Coach Carr took me aside and said, 'This team is depending on you, Brian. They're looking to you for leadership. So have fun out

there—but bring us back.' So we went out there and had some fun. First thing we did, we went right down the field, a sixty-seven-yard, eight-play drive that ended in a touchdown. After that, I was fine. And we won the game.

"To win, you have to be confident—and confidence comes from not taking things too seriously. When I play football, I know I can play this game. I never think, *What if I make a mistake?* I look at it this way: *It's just a game. I'm going to go out and have fun.* That takes the pressure off. Sure, you've gotta be serious about winning, and your teammates have to know you're serious—but at the same time, you have to have fun in order to be cool and calm and not get rattled in the pressure situations."

Fun! If you want to succeed, you just can't beat it. If you have fun at what you do, you just can't help being successful, because true success means doing what you love and loving what you do. Fact is, I'm having loads of fun right now. (Don't tell my publisher, but I can't believe he's actually paying me to write this book! This is *fun!*)

6. Manage your success well.

One of the smartest moves Reggie White ever made was when he married a beautiful young woman named Sara Copeland. They met when Sara was a college freshman at East Tennessee State in Knoxville and Reggie was a sophomore at the University of Tennessee. What Reggie didn't know at the time was that Sara was a *sixteen-year-old* college freshman—an indication of just how savvy and advanced Sara was for her age.

"Sara learned the value of a dollar at a very young age," Reggie told me. "When she was thirteen, she had an $11,000 bank account—money she had saved from working in her father's dry cleaning business. At twenty-one, after we'd been married for a year, she got her degree in marketing and management.

"I started playing professional football when I was twenty-one. The first check I got in the pros was a bonus check for $240,000. It kinda shocked me, 'cause I'd never seen that much money in my life! So I spent it kinda foolishly and I let people take advantage of me, 'cause I didn't know anything about money. At the end of my first year in the pros, I was close to going broke. What saved me was that I married Sara during my second year. She came in and rearranged everything. She was real businesslike and our money started increasing, so that we were not only able to be financially secure ourselves, but we were able to help others."

Thanks to the combination of Reggie's outstanding ability on the football field and Sara's intelligent handling of their finances, Reggie and Sara White have been able to give millions of dollars to improve the lives of people in need. Out of his own resources, he funded the Urban Hope Community Development Bank, which provides low-interest development loans, improving the lives of inner-city families.

It's one thing to be successful, but quite another thing to manage your success well. Many seemingly successful people are not as successful as they appear. They may wear $5,000 watches, drive a Jag or a Benz, and live on Millionaire's Row—but they are living from paycheck to paycheck. They look successful, but they are not managing their success well. As Thomas J. Stanley and William D. Danko observe in *The Millionaire Next Door*:

> Most people have it all wrong about wealth in America. Wealth is not the same as income. If you make a good income each year and spend it all, you are not getting wealthier. You are just living high. Wealth is what you accumulate, not what you spend.
>
> How do you become wealthy? Here, too, most people have it wrong. It is seldom luck or inheritance or advanced degrees or even intelligence that enables people to amass fortunes. Wealth is more often the result of a lifestyle of hard work, perseverance, planning, and most of all, self-discipline.[1]

In researching their book, Stanley and Danko found that wealthy people tend to have a number of factors in common. For example, wealthy people tend to live well below their means, often living in modest neighborhoods next door to people with a fraction as much wealth. They save and invest strategically and compulsively. They allocate considerable thought, time, and energy to building wealth. They come by their money by hard work, not inheritance—80 percent of millionaires, Stanley and Danko report, are "first-generation rich." The rich tend to marry once—and stay married (which helps conserve wealth). They are concerned with financial independence, not consumed with status and image.

Whether you are an entrepreneur, a sole proprietor, a manager, a corporate executive, or a supermarket stock boy, there are four simple rules for accumulating wealth. Follow these rules and you will become wealthy—in fact, you can't help but get wealthy. Ignore them, and no matter how big a paycheck you pull down, there's a good chance you'll reach retirement age with nothing to show for it but a stack of regrets.

The four rules are:

Rule No. 1. Beware of the warning signs of out-of-control finances.

The warning signs include:

- You find yourself unable to pay monthly bills on time.

- You find yourself unable to save on a regular basis.

- Your credit cards are maxed out and you can only make minimum payments on revolving debt.

- You find yourself trying to "borrow your way out of debt" with refinancing schemes and bill-consolidation loans.

- You and your partner argue about money and spending.

These warning signs mean it's time to get your spending under control, and maybe take an extra job to bring in more money.

Rule No. 2. Invest in "the miracle of compounding."

Albert Einstein once said, "Compounding is mankind's greatest invention because it allows for the reliable, systematic accumulation of wealth. The eighth wonder of the world is the miracle of compounding." Thanks to compound interest, a young person in America today, age twenty to twenty-five, has no excuse for not being a millionaire by retirement age. Anyone with a decent job and a measure of determination and self-discipline can do it. Here's how it works:

You make an investment that pays compound interest—that is, interest is computed not only on the original amount you invest, but also on the accumulated interest.

To determine how many years it takes for your investment to double in value, use "the Rule of 72." The formula is simple:

$$72 = R \times T$$

In this formula, R is the annual rate of return on investment (expressed in whole numbers, not decimals) and T is the number of years it takes the investment to double in value.

Let's say your investment earns 9 percent a year. According to the Rule of 72, R equals 9 (remember to use the whole number 9—not 0.09). So our formula reads $72 = 9 \times T$. What does T equal? To find out, you divide 72 by R (in this case, by 9) and you get 8. So T equals 8 years. This means that, at a compound rate of 9 percent, your investment doubles in value every eight years. So, for example, if you invest $5,000 at 9 percent and leave it there without ever adding another cent to your principal, here's what happens:

On day one, you have:	$5,000
After 8 years, you have:	$10,000
After 16 years, you have:	$20,000
After 24 years, you have:	$40,000
After 32 years, you have:	$80,000
After 40 years, you have:	$160,000
After 48 years, you have:	$320,000
After 56 years, you have:	$640,000
After 64 years, you have:	$1,280,000

With nothing more than patience, you've turned chump change into a millionaire's bankroll. That's the miracle of compounding.

Don't want to wait sixty-four years? Then simply put $5,000 away each year for thirty-four years, and presto! You're a millionaire!

Rule No. 3. Be frugal and self-disciplined.

Don't just live within your means—live *below* your means. To manage your success well, be content with spending less and investing more. Buy that bigger house or new car only when you can clearly afford it—don't buy in anticipation of being able to afford it down the road.

A good rule of thumb for home-buying: Never buy a home where the mortgage amount (that is, the purchase price less your down payment) is more than twice your annual income. So, for example, if you and your spouse/partner make a combined income of $100,000 and you have $50,000 for a down-payment, the maximum priced house you can afford is $250,000 ($250,000 minus $50,000 down-payment equals $200,000 or twice your combined income). The bank and your real estate agent will probably say you can afford a lot more—but they don't care that you won't be building up wealth while making payments on a $300,000 or $400,000 house.

You must be disciplined in your spending habits—but you must also be disciplined in your saving and investing habits. If you receive a regular paycheck, devote a portion of every paycheck to building up savings, investments, and assets. What if you are self-employed or get paid on commissions and don't receive a regular paycheck in a level amount? I hear that! I haven't received a regular paycheck in twenty-five years. My income is in the form of advances and royalty checks, and sometimes I go months between paychecks.

But there's a way to build wealth and manage your success even if you don't know how much income you'll receive from week to week, month to month. It's called "pay yourself first." Every time you get a check—from whatever source, in whatever amount, before you pay any bills or buy any groceries—sock away a certain amount (preferably 10 to 15 percent before taxes) in an interest-bearing investment as part of a wealth-building strategy.

Rule No. 4. Invest strategically and thoughtfully.

Become your own best financial expert. Read up on money and investing. Most of us pay at least 30 percent of our income to the IRS every year—but those who are good managers of their success know legitimate ways to pay only a fraction of that amount. And *please* don't tell me, "I don't pay taxes—I get a refund check every year." The money withheld from your paycheck is *your* money, whether you know it or not, even though it is snatched away before it reaches your outstretched hand. And there are legitimate ways to keep *more* of it.

One of the most productive strategies for managing your success is called "minimizing your realized income." In *The Millionaire Next Door*, Stanley and Danko use billionaire Ross Perot as an example of how to minimize realized income and dramatically reduce the tax bill. With a net worth of some $2.4 billion and an annual income of about $230 million, Perot paid only $19.5 million in taxes—or a mere 8.5 percent of his income. How did he do it? By investing heavily in tax-free municipal bonds, tax-sheltered real estate, and stocks with unrealized gains.

Stocks, for example, can be bought for, say, $10 a share and zoom in value to, say, $100 a share—but that is only a paper gain. It is not a *realized* gain until the stock is actually sold for that much. So a growing stock portfolio is a great way to increase your wealth without having to pay taxes on the increase until the stocks are actually converted into cash.

Stanley and Danko also point out that while the typical American household pays the equivalent of 11.6 percent of its net worth each year in taxes, billionaire Perot paid only 0.8 percent of his net worth in taxes.[2] Should we rant and rave about the injustice of having to pay fourteen and a half times more of our net worth to the taxman than Ross Perot? No. He's just playing by the rules. You can play by those same rules if you do your homework, manage your success, and invest as wisely as a billionaire.

7. Manage your personal and family life well.

Success ultimately means little if you have no one to share it with— and that means *family*. Building a loving, functional family takes work, time, and attention. I'm not saying divorce is the end of everything. I personally know a number of people who have made a new start after a divorce, and they are making a rousing success of their new life. I also know there are times when a marriage can be so bad that you need to get out and get on with your life.

But all too many divorces take place because somebody got bored or had unrealistic expectations or was simply too immature to work through the normal passages of an otherwise salvageable relationship. Divorce is especially hard on children—they get caught up in the nonsense and lunacy that their parents generate, and their lives are torn right down the middle. That's certainly the worst of it—but there's more.

Divorce is unbelievably expensive.

Divorce devastates wealth, health, and happiness.

Divorce sabotages success.

Fact is, marriage is good for success. According to John Hinderaker of the Center of the American Experiment, married people tend to earn more and accumulate more wealth than single people, divorced people, and unmarried couples living together. Married people can merge their incomes while cutting expenses. Married people statistically tend to be healthier, which means greater productivity and fewer medical expenses. Married people tend to live longer—and that means they have more time to work and invest and enjoy the fruits of their success.[3] So if you want to be successful, manage your personal and family life well.

Shared, not stockpiled

These, then, are the seven essential rules for a successful life:

1. Define what success means to you.

2. Dream big dreams.

3. Keep faith with your dreams.

4. Be the best you can be.

5. Stay loose and have fun.

6. Manage your success well.

7. Manage your personal and family life well.

Nothing complicated here—just simple, practical, *transforming* principles. Follow these steps on a daily basis, and you will experience a level of success that satisfies the soul—especially if you keep in mind the true aim and meaning of success. Genuine success means much more than merely becoming rich or famous. It means being able to do something noble and meaningful with our achievements. The only way to make success meaningful is to *share* our success—gratefully, compassionately, and generously—with those around us, with people who are less fortunate, with a needy community, with a hurting world. Success is to be shared, not stockpiled.

So how about you? I know you're going to be successful in whatever you commit yourself to. The bigger question is this: How will you invest your success in making the world a better place?

3

How Can I Increase My Luck?

Over the years we've been married, my wife, Debbie, has won a lot of radio contests—cash prizes, a shopping spree at Linens N' Things, dinner for four at a terrific restaurant, a Honey Baked Ham, a trip for four to Disneyland (including airfare and hotel), and more. Winning these contests doesn't change your lifestyle in a huge way, but it's a lot of fun.

I've always marveled at Debbie's luck. When we were first married, we used to play cards a lot, especially pinochle. Over a run of a hundred games, even the worst pinochle player in the world is bound to win at least once, right? But I have never beaten Debbie at pinochle in my life. I mean that literally: Not once! So where does her luck at cards come from?

"What luck?" she replied coyly when I asked. "That's skill."

"Skill, huh?" I queried. "Well, then, what about all those contests? Was that skill, too? C'mon, how do you do it? How come I never win anything?"

"Did you ever enter a contest?"

"Uh, no," said I, rather sheepishly.

"Well, there you are."

At that moment, a light came on in my darkened belfry. Aha! If you want to *win* the contest, you must *enter* the contest! So, about six months ago as I write these words, I entered a radio station contest—and I won five hundred dollars! Absolutely true!

In the process, I learned the first rule of increasing your luck: *Enter the contest, stupid!* In fact, as I've examined the lives of many so-called "lucky" people, I've learned that there are a lot of simple, practical things we can all do to increase our luck in life.

Demystifying luck

What is luck?

A lot of people think of luck in mystical, almost religious terms. Luck, they believe, is a powerful force that shapes our destiny. Some study the omens and signs that supposedly indicate whether luck is moving *for* them or *against* them. They check their horoscope before getting out of bed. They wear or collect Buddha amulets, crosses, Saint Christopher medals, Egyptian ankhs, crystals, polished stones, lodestones, elk teeth, rabbits' feet, alligator feet, buckeyes, four-leaf clovers, pyramids, garlic, horseshoes, scarab beetle amulets, unicorn amulets, and wishbones. They invoke lucky numbers when buying lottery tickets or playing the roulette wheel. They walk into a casino and play a few slot machines—"just to see how my luck is running"—before going on to the bigger games. They avoid the number thirteen, black cats, broken mirrors, and other harbingers of "bad luck."

To such people, the world is a magical place ruled by that elusive goddess, "Lady Luck." She may help you or hurt you, but she can never be controlled. She can be influenced, however—*if* you know the right numbers and incantations and have the right charms in your mojo bag.

Other people would say that luck is not a force; it is simply random chance. Stuff happens. Good stuff. Bad stuff. You can't predict it, avert it, control it, or even influence it. Luck is nothing but the unpredictable occurrence of haphazard events. A random roll of the dice, that's all there is to it. I tend to fall into this camp. Experience tells me that the natural world we live in is ordered and rational, though unpredictable. If luck is a "force," then it is the "force" of chance and probability.

Even so, I believe we *can* influence our luck. We can take deliberate steps to become luckier people. Whether we see luck as a mysterious force or sheer blind chance, we can actually *make our own luck* to some degree. No, we can't ward off every disastrous event. Sometimes bad luck just comes blundering into our lives through no fault of our own. But I have observed again and again that the luckiest people in the world are those who take responsibility for their own destiny.

You may not have been "born lucky," but you don't have to play the cards you were dealt. You *can* improve your hand. Here's how.

Make your own luck

"I know what you're thinking," growled Inspector Harry Callahan (Clint Eastwood), waving the muzzle of his .357 Magnum long-barrel in the face of a cornered felon. " 'Did he fire six shots or only five?' Well, to tell you the truth, in all this excitement I kind of lost track myself. You've got to ask yourself one question, 'Do I feel lucky?' Well, do you, punk?" The punk, a would-be holdup man in the movie *Dirty Harry*, clearly did not feel lucky. He had no reason to. He had made his own luck that day— all of it bad. But if you follow these simple steps, the next time someone asks you, "Do you feel lucky?" you'll be able to say, "You bet I do!"

1. Be sociable.

Make friends and contacts. Don't wait for good fortune to come to you—go out and meet it with a broad smile and a warm handshake. You've probably heard this complaint: "I don't know how she does it! She's always in the right place at the right time! She always gets the sale, the deal, the promotion ahead of everybody else!" More than likely, she makes an *effort* to be in the right place at the right time. Lucky people position themselves for good fortune by being proactive, gregarious, and sociable. As a result, the word gets around, so when a sale is to be made, a deal is to be done, or a better job opens up, the first person everyone thinks of is Mr. or Ms. Lucky.

When you build a network of relationships, you create a luck-friendly environment. Example: Only a few of the nearly fifty books I've written have been sold on spec to an editor who didn't know me. In almost every case, I either knew the editor or knew someone who knew the editor. You may say, "Oh, right! It's not *what* you know but *who* you know!" No. It's *both*. You have to be good at what you do *and* you have to let people know you are good at what you do. If you are good and gregarious, you'll get lucky. If you are good but unknown, or if you are lousy and gregarious, you will strike out. It's as simple as that.

In his 1977 book *The Luck Factor*, Max Gunther tells the story of how actor Kirk Douglas got his start in Hollywood. Shortly before the beginning of World War II, Douglas was one of hundreds of struggling, obscure actors in New York. He lived in a cramped little room in Greenwich Village, waited tables at Schrafft's, scrambled for bit parts on Broadway, but got nowhere in his career. Still, he was convivial, charming, and outgoing, and he made a lot of friends among the aspiring actors and actresses he hung out with, including a beautiful young ingenue named Betty Jean Perske.

After Pearl Harbor, Kirk Douglas joined the Navy, seeing action in the Pacific. When he returned, he found that Betty Jean had become a box-office sensation playing opposite Humphrey Bogart in *To Have and Have Not*, but her name was no longer Betty Jean Perske. All the world knew her as Lauren Bacall. She put Kirk Douglas in touch with Hollywood producer Hal Wallis, whom she knew through her friendship with Bogart. Hal Wallis then cast Kirk Douglas in a supporting role with Barbara Stanwick in *The Strange Love of Martha Ivers*, and Douglas was on his way to stardom.

"Your own luck depends on other people's luck," Douglas recalls. "It's crazy! ... Oh, sure, I guess I had some kind of talent. But if it hadn't been for this Lauren Bacall fluke, where would the talent have gone? Dozens of my friends back then had talent too, but you don't see their names in movies today. They didn't have the luck." Or, perhaps, they didn't *make* their own luck. Kirk Douglas made his luck by knowing a lot of "unknown" people, and when one of those "unknowns" became a star, so did he.[1]

A friendly, outgoing personality is a lucky asset to have. "But," you may say, "I'm not like that! I'm shy and I'm tongue-tied!" I know what you mean. I'm a naturally shy person myself. But I'm learning to overcome it—and people who knew me years ago would tell you I've changed a lot over the years. Nobody is doomed to be unlucky just because he is shy. Some are fortunate enough to be born with a bold, outgoing personality, but the rest of us can *choose* to be bold and outgoing, and we can make our own luck.

2. Be prepared.

Opportunities come to us all, but if we are not prepared to seize those opportunities, our luck will pass us by. Lucky people are ready to act at a moment's notice. They have disciplined and prepared themselves for their big chance.

One of the luckiest quarterbacks in NFL history is Bob Griese, who led the Miami Dolphins to victory in Super Bowl VII, capping the only undefeated season in NFL history. But there was a moment during one particular game that season when Bob didn't feel so lucky.

In the first quarter of a home game against the San Diego Chargers,

Bob dropped back to pass and saw two linemen, Deacon Jones and Ron East, bullrushing straight for him. He got the ball away, but he paid for it big-time. East hit him low, breaking Bob's leg and dislocating his ankle. Coach Don Shula sent in backup quarterback Earl Morrall, and the Dolphins pulled out an emotional win, 24 to 10.

For the next couple of months, Bob hobbled up and down the sidelines on crutches, his leg in a cast, while his team won game after game without him. Throughout his recovery, he kept up with team meetings and workouts, keeping his head

> "Don't wait for good fortune to come to you—go out and meet it with a broad smile and a warm handshake."

in the game. As soon as the doctor okayed it, he began throwing the ball, taking laps, and taking part in the workouts.

"I kept up mentally and physically," Bob told me, "because when Shula needed me, I wanted to be ready. The worst thing in the world is when the coach turns to you and says, 'Okay, you're in the game,' and you go in and drop the ball because you weren't prepared. You never know when your chance is going to come, but you have to prepare as if you're going to start every game. It's tough to go through it week after week, saying, 'I'm ready to play,' but it doesn't happen. After a while, you're tempted to let down. But you can't let down. You have to be ready."

On New Year's Eve 1972, the Dolphins went to Pittsburgh for the AFC championship game. Bob Griese was suited up and ready to play, but Coach Don Shula started Earl Morrall instead. The Dolphins' offense struggled during the first half, and the score was tied at 7 at halftime. In the locker room, Shula asked Bob if he was prepared to play.

"I'm ready," he replied.

"You start the second half," said Shula.

The second half was a tough, seesaw contest, but by the end, Bob Griese and the Dolphins had won it, 21 to 17. From there, it was on to Super Bowl VII, where Bob led the Dolphins to a world championship, beating the Washington Redskins 14 to 7—a perfect 17 and 0 season.

Would you call Bob Griese lucky because he was able to come back from a serious injury and lead the Dolphins to a Super Bowl victory and an undefeated season? Yeah, I would, because Bob Griese *made his own luck.* He worked hard. He trained. Even when he was on the sidelines, hobbling on crutches, his head and his heart were in the game. And when his opportunity came, he was *prepared.*

3. Be positive.

The most positive person I've ever met is Patrick Livingston Murphy Williams, former general manager and now executive vice president with the Orlando Magic organization. Pat Williams is so optimistic, it's scary. If you phone his voice-mail, you have to wait for about a minute or so while Pat's recorded voice reels out his latest motivational quotation or joke of the week—and you won't mind a bit because it's worth it. When we talk, he has a lot of different names for me: James, Big Fella, Coach—though why he calls *me* Coach, I dunno. He's the guy who's always motivating me! "To have a happy, positive, joy-filled life," he once told me, "you have to feast on today, you have to pig out on today, you have to absolutely suck the marrow from the bones of today. This is your moment. Live it. Use it. Devour it."

When I was assisting Pat on his highly successful motivational book, *Go For the Magic,* he shared this story with me: "A few years ago," he said, "I was invited to play in Charles Barkley's Celebrity Golf Tournament at one of the Disney courses in Orlando. I have to tell you, I'm the world's biggest duffer. I have a wonderful short game. Unfortunately, it's off the tee.

"Also in this tournament was a fella by the name of Michael Jordan. He's a great golfer, and I've heard he plays a fair game of basketball, too. He's also a great needler—an opinionated guy who will shower you with his opinions like a grenade showers you with shrapnel. And wouldn't you know it? His foursome was right behind mine! As we were moving along, I looked back and there was Michael, just one hole behind us—and gaining! Everything slowed down around the thirteenth hole, a par three, up on a hill, shooting down over some water. We had to wait for the foursome ahead of us, and by the time I got to the tee, Michael's foursome had descended upon us, along with his media entourage.

"I had not hit a ball solidly all day, and suddenly I was surrounded by TV cameras and watchful eyes, and I had to produce a shot under scrutiny! And the worst of it was Michael Jordan himself, needling me the whole time I was trying to muster my concentration. I mean, you talk about sweaty palms and prayer! *Lord,* I said, *if I can just hit one ball well, I'll be satisfied!*

"I settled down, planted my feet, visualized a long, straight, sailing drive—then I took my shot. It was amazing. That ball climbed into the sky, high, straight, and true. There was total silence all around as the crowd watched that ball go. For a moment, even Michael was at a loss for words! The ball landed on the green, just a nice little putt from the hole. As I started down the hill toward the green, I could hear Michael's voice: 'Hey, Pat! It's easy to see *you* don't spend much time at the office!' That little jab from Michael Jordan was the finest compliment my modest golfing skills have ever received!

"I got down to the green and totally blew the putt. But I couldn't have cared less—I had made the one shot that really counted."

Positive people attract good luck—but not, I'm convinced, through any mystical or supernatural means. A positive mental attitude enables people to perform better by believing in themselves. They are able to imagine their successes—just as Pat "visualized a long, straight, sailing drive." And then positive people make their visions come true. Confidence, enthusiasm, and a positive attitude help to steady us, energize us, and focus us for the task at hand. And when we approach our challenges with an inner peace and confidence, we just can't help being lucky.

4. Be bold.

Unlucky people are passive people. "Take no chances," they say, "and you won't get hurt." But lucky people are bold, they demonstrate pluck and initiative, and they take responsibility for designing their own lives. Lucky people don't wait for things to happen; they *make* things happen. Here's another great Pat Williams story, which he told me as we were working on his autobiography, *Ahead of the Game*.

In 1995, as Pat was going through the process of a painful divorce, he attended a two-day Orlando Magic retreat called Magic University—a series of seminars, workshops, and brainstorming sessions held at Disney World's Pleasure Island. "I sit down," Pat recalls, "and wait for the seminar to begin. I'm fighting off drowsiness and wondering how I'm going to get through the next few hours when I look up and this pert, five-foot-three blonde comes out and launches right into her presentation. From her first word, I knew this woman was unique. Her name was Ruth Hanchey."

After the seminar, Pat boldly struck up a conversation with her and walked her to her car. His own car was nearby, so he grabbed a copy of

Go For the Magic out of the trunk and signed it for her. As she drove away, Pat said to himself, *Wow! There goes a fascinating woman!* Over the next few months, they exchanged phone calls and occasionally met for lunch or dinner.

With the end of 1996 came the divorce decree, and Pat felt sad but relieved. The loss of his first marriage had been terribly painful—but at last the ordeal was over and he could get on with his life. And he wanted his life to include Ruth. After the divorce was finalized, Ruth asked Pat, "Where do we go from here?"

Pat had been reading a lot of books about relationships, and several of the books warned against rushing into a new relationship right after a divorce. So he replied, "I'm not sure where we go from here, Ruth, but the books say I should take time to let the emotional dust settle."

"Well, how long does this dust-settling thing take?" asked Ruth.

"According to the book, about two years—"

"Two years!" Ruth exclaimed. "Well, if that's the way you want it—"

"After that," Pat told me, "I would call Ruth and she didn't seem as cordial as before." Time passed, and she grew increasingly more distant. Finally, she called and said, "Pat, I've met a man...."

"A chill went through me," Pat recalls. "I knew right then how I really felt about Ruth—and I had let her get away!"

A few weeks later, Pat learned that Ruth was flying to Orlando to conduct a seminar. He called and offered to meet her plane, which was arriving at ten that night.

"Pat, please don't come," Ruth replied. "I can't handle this right now."

And here is where *boldness* comes into the picture. "Ruth had made it clear that she didn't want to see me," Pat explains. "So I had a decision to make: Should I abide by her wishes—or disregard them? I figured, *What have I got to lose? As things stand, I've lost her already—so how could I make things worse by showing up?* So I went."

Pat arrived at the airport and found that Ruth's plane was running four hours late because of winter weather. Now what? Should he go back home and forget it—or sit out the next four hours in the airport? He decided to stay. So he found a booth seat at the closed and shuttered Burger King across from Gate 82 and took a snooze. Sometime later, he woke up, checked his watch—and it was almost two in the morning.

"I sat up," Pat told me. "A group of beleaguered-looking passengers was filing off a Delta arrival. I waited—and there she was, pulling her suitcase on a little cart, looking like she had just survived a very long day. I stepped up behind her and followed her, and I tell you, Jim, my heart was pounding like a jackhammer! Soon I was beside her, and we walked along like that—and for a few steps, Ruth was completely unaware of me. I kept thinking, *What will she do? What will she think? What will she say?* All of a sudden, it seemed she sensed me there alongside her. She stopped in her tracks and looked at me with an expression of shock.

"Well, that was the moment of truth. She was either going to throw her arms around me or she was going to tell me off but good. And there was a long moment where it seemed it could have gone either way. But then her eyes lit up and she hugged me and said, 'Pat! I'm so glad you came!' "

Pat offered to drive Ruth to her hotel, and she accepted. They arrived at the Marriott International Drive at 2:30 A.M., but they didn't get out. Instead, they sat in the car and talked straight through the night. As the sun was coming up, Pat proposed to Ruth—and Ruth accepted. Then they pulled out their Franklin Planners, compared schedules, and settled on a wedding date. They had a beautiful lakeside wedding, and are now living their storybook romance as man and wife—

But it all hinged on a decision Pat made to boldly go to the Orlando airport late one night after Ruth told him to stay away. On such pivotal decisions do our lives and our luck depend.

5. Reduce your exposure to risk.

Lucky people take risks—but they take *calculated* risks, not stupid gambles. They are not just optimistic—they are *cautiously* optimistic. Lucky people calculate the odds, avoid unnecessary risk, and never take a sucker bet.

Writing in *Men's Health*, Joe Kita talks about the risks and rewards we all face in life—and about how to turn the odds in our favor so as to decrease the risks and increase the rewards. For example, the odds of getting some form of cancer during your lifetime are about fifty-fifty—but you can reduce your risk of cancer death by more than half by simply avoiding all forms of tobacco and secondhand smoke, limiting sun exposure, limiting alcohol intake to less than two drinks a day, limiting dietary fat and controlling weight, eating high-fiber foods, and getting regular cancer screenings.

Kita noted that your lifetime odds of being struck by lightning are one in 10,456—not a risk that should particularly trouble your sleep. But in case you are worried about being zapped during a thunderstorm, you can decrease your odds by avoiding open areas, staying away from isolated trees or tall structures, getting inside a car or building, avoiding bodies of water, and keeping your hands off metal objects like umbrellas and nine-irons. Also, stay out of Florida from July to September—that's the riskiest time of year in the riskiest state of the union for lightning strikes. If you feel your skin tingle and your hair stand up straight, look out—there's a thunderbolt up there with your name on it. So run to the nearest building or crouch low. Any other advice? "The protective effect of prayer has not been scientifically calculated," says Kita, "but in a situation like this, go for it."

Your lifetime odds of being murdered are one in 140—but your luck improves dramatically—*if*! For example, if you move out of Washington, D.C. (where the annual murder rate is one in 1,330) to Mesa, Arizona (one in 33,334). Or if you quit that taxi-driving job. Or if you stay sober (nearly half of all murder victims were drinking at the time). And if you avoid Lesotho, a country with a one in 710 annual murder rate.

You have a one in seventy-five lifetime risk of dying in a car crash, but you better your odds by observing the laws regarding speed, alcohol, and lap/shoulder belts—that's just common sense. But here's an interesting factoid: Staying married decreases your odds of dying in a crash—divorced men are 400 percent more likely to be traffic fatalities than married men. Don't ask me why. You also better your luck by driving an Acura Legend, a Plymouth Voyager or a Lincoln Town Car—and avoiding Corvettes and convertibles.

Kita says that the odds that a gambler will make money over the long haul are one in 5,000. You can improve your luck by sticking with the near even-money games like blackjack, craps, and roulette. But state lotteries are for chumps. The odds of winning the California lottery are one in 18 million; the New York lottery, one in 25.8 million; the seventeen-state Powerball jackpot, one in 55 million. To put that into perspective, your odds of winning any of these jackpots are about the same as the odds of being struck and killed by an airplane falling out of the sky (a one in 25 million annual risk). In fact, you have a much greater chance of dying by falling out of your bed or chair (one in 513,142 annually) than you do of winning the lottery. You want to get lucky? Then avoid sucker bets. Avoid *foolish* risks and take only *calculated* risks.[2]

6. Be careful.

In *The Luck Factor*, Max Gunther tells the story of Isadora Duncan, a flamboyant dancer who helped found the modern dance movement. Duncan had a flair for the dramatic in everything she did, as exemplified by the long flowing scarves she always wore. Gunther says that one of Duncan's friends, cosmetics entrepreneur Helena Rubinstein, considered adopting Duncan's dramatic style, but worried that those scarves would get caught in doors. Rubinstein's instincts were good. In 1927, Isadora Duncan was killed when the scarf she had tied around her neck got tangled in the wire-spoked wheel of the open roadster she was riding in. She was killed instantly when the scarf snapped her neck.

Those who knew Isadora Duncan called her "accident prone." But how can that be? As a dancer, she certainly wasn't clumsy—she was renowned for her grace and agility. But she was continually stubbing her toes and cutting her fingers—and once she even fell through a hole in the deck of a cruise ship. Fact is, she was *careless*—careless in every aspect of her life. Besides her many careless injuries, she was continually in legal and financial trouble because she was astoundingly careless with money, documents, and passports. Isadora Duncan was an unlucky woman because she made her own bad luck.

Lucky people plan for calamities and contingencies. They ponder worst-case scenarios. They respect Murphy's Law. They prepare themselves so that when something goes wrong, they know what to do to make it right again. Lucky people are *careful* people.

7. Be flexible.

Lucky people roll with the punches. They make adjustments when conditions change. My friend Barry McGuire knows how to be flexible. If you're from my generation, you remember Barry—he sang the biggest hit record of 1965, "Eve of Destruction." I remember exactly where I was and what I was doing when I first heard that song—it had that kind of impact on my twelve-year-old soul. The way that song came about is a case study in the wildly unpredictable workings of luck.

At the time, Barry had recently ended a successful run with the folk group The New Christy Minstrels and was working on his first solo album. "Eve of Destruction" was one of the cuts on that album.

"'Eve of Destruction' was recorded in one take," Barry told me, "under kind of weird circumstances. We'd already recorded two songs, and the third one wasn't coming out right. We only had about thirty minutes left in the recording session. The producer said, 'This one sounds too much like the first one. Let's do something else.' I said, 'Let's do that Phil Sloan tune.' So I pulled out the lyrics to 'Eve of Destruction'—the paper was all crumpled from being in my pocket for about a week. I smoothed out the wrinkles and we wrote down the chords on pieces of a brown paper bag from somebody's lunch. We ran through the song twice, so everybody knew it, then they rolled tape and we did it again.

"Well, they were playing and I was singing, reading the words off this piece of wrinkly paper. I got to the part that goes, 'Well, my blood's so mad, feels like coagulatin' —and I lost my place. So while I'm looking for the line, I go, 'Ahhhhh!' and then I slide right into that line, 'Ahhhhh, you can't twist the truth.' And after the song came out, people would hear that line and say, 'Man, you really get into the message of that song! You really sound angry!' Well, I *was* angry! I was mad because I couldn't find the words! I wanted to rerecord the vocal track, but the producer said, 'We're out of time. We'll come back next week and do the vocal track again.'"

For some unknown reason, the engineer made a vinyl demo from the tape, which went to the producer's office. By pure serendipity, a music promoter stopped by the producer's office, picked up the demo, and played it at a backyard birthday party for the daughter of the program director of KFWB, L.A.'s blowtorch rock station. The kids at the birthday party went crazy over the song, demanding that it be played again and again. The program director told the promoter, "Find the producer of this record! Tell him if this song can be mixed down and released by Monday morning, KFWB will play it as the Pick-to-Hit record of the week!"

The producer tried to reach Barry to bring him back into the studio to produce a cleaned-up version of "Eve of Destruction," but Barry was out partying. So the producer took the tapes he had, brought in some studio musicians to add backup vocals, did a quick mix-down, and actually got records pressed and in the stores by Monday morning—with Barry's frustrated growl still on the vocal track. The first Barry knew of the song's release was when his phone rang at seven o'clock on Monday morning and the president of Dunhill Records told him, "Hey, McGuire, turn your radio on to KFWB."

Within days, "Eve of Destruction" had exploded to Number One. It seemed that every radio station in the country was either playing "Eve of Destruction" or banning it—and banning the song was even better for sales than playing it!

Before "Eve of Destruction," Barry was part of a loose-knit L.A. coffeehouse fraternity—a group of unknown, soon-to-be-discovered rock legends that included John Sebastian, David Crosby, Roger McGuinn of The Byrds, and The Mamas and the Papas. In fact, one of the M&P's most famous songs, "Creeque Alley," talks about those days when McGuinn and McGuire were just a-gettin' higher, and no one was gettin' fat except Mama Cass. After "Eve of Destruction," Barry's life changed in a big way. He moved to a huge house in the Hollywood hills. He did TV appearances. He tried acting, appearing opposite James Coburn in *The President's Analyst*.

He quickly went to work on a second album to follow up the success of "Eve of Destruc-tion." His backup group for the second album was the then-unknown Mamas and the Papas. In fact, the M&Ps' lead singer and songwriter, John Phillips, wrote a pow-erful new song that

> "Lucky people plan for calamities and contingencies. They ponder worst-case scenarios. They respect Murphy's Law. They prepare themselves so that when something goes wrong, they know what to do to make it right again."

Barry recorded for his new album. Barry sang the lead vocal on that song, and the M&Ps sang backup. As a favor to his friends, Barry introduced The Mamas and the Papas to his producer at Dunhill, who promptly signed them to record an album of their own.

A few days after Barry recorded the song, John Phillips approached Barry and asked to have the song back—Phillips wanted it for The Ma-mas and the Papas debut album. "Well, sure, John, you can have it," said Barry. "You wrote it. It's your song." So they took the recording Barry had made, stripped out Barry's vocal track, laid in a new lead vocal by Phillips, and released the record. That song was called "California Dreamin'," and it became a huge Number One hit for The Mamas and the Papas, launching their recording career. If you listen closely to that recording, you can faintly hear Barry's gravel-road baritone in that song.

Would Barry's McGuire's version of "California Dreamin'" have been a huge hit? Absolutely. It was virtually the same recording that put The Mamas and the Papas on the map. As it turned out, Barry never had another chart-busting megahit like "Eve of Destruction." So was it bad luck that Barry passed up the chance to make "California Dreamin'" his own hit song?

"No," Barry told me. "Fact is, I'm *glad* I never got another hit. John Phillips probably saved my life when he asked for that song back. My lifestyle was one of complete self-indulgence and self-destruction. If I had gotten another hit like 'Eve of Destruction,' I would have been able to finance my death in high style. I would have ended up just like Jimi Hendrix or Jim Morrison."

That's what I mean about being flexible. Good luck doesn't always mean fame and fortune. Some people are killed by fame and fortune. Their success is their misfortune. It takes a lot of maturity to see that what looks like good luck to most people can actually be a curse. So when "bad luck" comes your way, be flexible. Learn from it. Grow wise from it. Your "bad luck" could be the luckiest thing that ever happened to you.

There's no real mystery to this thing called luck. We plan out our lives, all neat and orderly—then Lady Luck comes along and tells us what's *really* going to happen. Unlucky people moan and groan and surrender to their fate. Lucky people simply make new plans.

So good luck to you! As my Irish forebears used to say, "May your pockets be heavy and your heart be light, / May good luck pursue you each morning and night."

And may the luck you wish for be the luck you *make*.

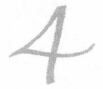

How Can I Put More Time in My Day?

Hold out your hands. *Both* hands. Careful, don't drop it! I just put $86,400 in your hands. That's right. It's all yours, a free gift. What's the catch, you ask? Well, there's just one *little* catch. You have to spend it all today. That's right, you can spend it any way you like, but at the end of the day, I take back whatever's left.

But tomorrow, you get the same deal—$86,400, all yours, spend it any way you like, and at the end of the day, it's gone. Next day, same thing. And the day after that and the day after that, for as long as you live.

Sound like a good deal to you?

Well, by now you've probably figured out that I was only making an analogy. No, I'm not *really* giving away money to everyone who reads this book. Fact is, you've already got the same deal I described—only you don't get 86,400 *dollars*. You get something even more valuable. You get 86,400 *seconds* to spend as you please. That's how many seconds there are in a day. What are you going to do with them?

Well, you can spend them, invest them, or waste them. You can use those seconds to move closer to your goals. You can use them to improve your mind. You can invest them in a rewarding relationship or in building your career. You can spend them zoned out in front of a TV set. You can use them for eating, sleeping, thinking, reading, conversing, working, praying, exercising, helping others, making love, or getting drunk. It's entirely up to you. But at the end of the day, all of those 86,400 seconds are gone, and you can never get them back.

It's your life. It's your choice. And it's your loss if you don't use your time wisely.

Not a moment to waste

People say time is money. I say time is life.

When you pick up a paycheck, you are making a life-and-death transaction. You are trading a chunk of your life, your finite mortal existence, for a medium of exchange called money. Over the span of your lifetime, you will have only a certain number of heartbeats, a certain number of seconds, a certain number of years. When they're gone, they're gone.

Ever hear someone say, "I'm just killing time"? What is he really saying? "I'm just killing *myself*." Because time is all you have, and when it's gone, you're dead. When you kill time, you kill yourself, moment by moment, second by second, a little bit at a time.

"People with a keen sense of the preciousness of time are a valuable resource," my friend Pat Williams once told me. "They are the leaders, the go-getters, the entrepreneurial spirits. They're the people you can count on to get the job done. People who understand the value of one tick of the clock are the ones who make the world a better place."

Pat, who is executive vice president of the Orlando Magic franchise of the NBA, offers this analogy from the business of basketball. "In our game," he said, "time is everything. You've got four twelve-minute quarters to get the job done—forty-eight minutes to shoot more baskets than the other guy. As soon as the ball is inbounded, the shot clock starts ticking. You've got just twenty-four seconds to shoot, or the ball turns over. And you don't have the luxury of taking a nice, leisurely shot. Usually, you're double-teamed, and you've got to find some way to force the shot while that clock is ticking down. It's not easy—but there's no finer feeling in the world than beating the buzzer and making the pressure shot. It's the same way in life."

Life is precious, time is irreplaceable. Maybe you can afford to waste it, but I can't. I know that life is short. I don't have a moment to waste.

The myth of "when I have more time"

I wish I had a dollar for every time I've heard someone say, "Someday, when I have more time..." I used to say that a lot myself. But now I know better. I'm never going to have more time than I have right now.

For some reason, people always think that there is a magical "someday" out there when they will be less busy, when there will be fewer responsibilities and demands on their time, when the pace of life will slow down to a leisurely crawl—some mythical someday "when I have more time." But if you truly want to make your dreams come true, you can't wait until "someday." You have to do it *now*.

My friend Phil Brewer, who is a counselor and leadership trainer, told me about a trip he took to Europe in 1977. "I went to Switzerland and interviewed several writers and thinkers, including Paul Tournier, the great Swiss psychiatrist," he told me. "And there is one statement Dr. Tournier made that had a profound impact on my life. He said to me in his wonderful French-accented English, 'People are always looking for the right time and the perfect place to write, to paint, to accomplish some goal. They say, "I have to be in the mountains, I have to be on the coast, everything must be just so." But if you look at all the great achievements of history, you will see that they have largely been done in cold, cramped, unpicturesque conditions. Look where all the great people and all the great achievements have come from, and you see that they always seem to come from deprived situations.'

"Those words hit me right between the eyes. It took me years to fully absorb the great truth that Dr. Tournier had given to me. I'm still absorbing it. I think he saw in me a perfectionist streak that so often keeps me from starting a project until 'just the right moment.' I want a cup of coffee, but I want to drink it on the beach in Maui. The point is this: If you're going to write the Great American Novel, then write it. Don't put it off until everything's just so. *Do it*, and do it *now*."

Six practical tips for putting more time in your day

Effective time management begins with personal responsibility. You and I are each responsible for the way we invest our time. We can't expect anyone else to organize our schedules or remind us of our goals. You own your own day, and I own mine. You and you alone are responsible for how you invest your time—or how you squander it.

Here, then, are some tips for taking charge of your day in such a way that—like magic!—it will actually seem you are putting more time into your day.

1. Organize and prioritize.

In order to achieve your most important goals, you must *prioritize your time*. First order of business: Make a list. And whatever you do, *don't lose that list*! Call it a "Things To Do" list or a "Priorities" list. I keep mine on my computer, and it's the first thing I see when I boot up in the morning. Every time I think of a new priority to be added, I just add it to the list. I break my list down into three categories:

Priority 1. Cherished dreams and goals.
Priority 2. Urgencies and emergencies.
Priority 3. Marginalia and nonessentials.

Let's take a closer look at each of these priorities and how to manage them.

Priority 1: Cherished dreams and goals. This is the category where you list such things as that dream house you want to build or the novel you want to write—whatever it is that will take you where you want to be in life. Priority 1 items are things that are essential, but not necessarily urgent. It's where you put your grand dreams, your hopes for the future, the things that you truly want in life, but which tend to get crowded out by things that are less essential but more urgent.

Priority 2: Urgencies and emergencies. This is the category where you list the things that need to get done right away, the stuff that keeps you out of the jailhouse or the poorhouse or the doghouse. Like preparing for that presentation at the office next week. Or renewing your driver's license. Or filing your 1040. Or scheduling that root canal. Or cleaning out one of the stalls of your three-car garage so you can put your car away at night.

Doing Priority 2 stuff doesn't really enrich your life or move you toward your dreams and goals—but *not* getting your Priority 2 stuff done can really make your life a living hell. It's the work you need to get done—or else. These chores may not enhance your life, *but they are always urgent.*

Priority 3: Marginalia and nonessentials. This is the category where you list things that need to get done, but which are medium to low priority. Often these tasks are the smallest and most easily accomplished, like "E-mail Joe and Mandy" or "Take down Xmas lights" or "Call Congressman Fogbottom, give him a piece of my mind."

Once you have your list of priorities, allocate time accordingly. If you know you have nine hours to spend today, then allocate the appropriate amount of time to each of your priorities. You can allocate it in any way that makes sense to you. Personally, if I had nine hours to divvy up, I'd probably do it this way: five hours to Priority 1 tasks; three hours to Priority 2 tasks; and one hour to Priority 3 tasks. Priority 1 tasks are the things I most want to get done; Priority 2 tasks are the things I've gotta get done; and Priority 3 tasks are things that will pile up and annoy me if they don't eventually get done. Here's a simple plan for attacking these priorities:

Tackle Priority 1 tasks first. This is what the time management experts will tell you, and it seems rather obvious. However, I have a tendency to procrastinate in the face of big, overwhelming Priority 1 tasks, so I sometimes start my day with one or two simple Priority 3 tasks, like writing a short e-mail to a friend. That gives me the good feeling of scratching one more task off my list. Then it's easier to switch over to the bigger, more imposing Priority 1 tasks.

> *"You and you alone are responsible for how you invest your time—or how you squander it."*

Break down big, intimidating projects into bite-size, nonthreatening chunks. For example, instead of putting "Write the Great American Novel" on your list, break it down into smaller component tasks: "Outline plot," "Write character sketches," "Research background and setting," "Write Chapter 1," and so forth.

Group together activities that are logically related, and do them in batches for maximum efficiency. Do one three-stop shopping trip instead of three trips. If you have a half dozen letters to write, write 'em in a row. Maximize effectiveness by minimizing transition time, decision time, and down time.

Organize tasks by segmenting them on a timetable. Set high but reasonable expectations (if your expectations are too high, you set yourself up for discouragement). Things get done faster when you shoot for a deadline.

Don't procrastinate. Start *now*. Do one thing at a time, finish it completely, then move to the next item.

Organizing your priorities is essential to putting more time into your day. A surgeon was once asked what he would do if he only had five minutes to perform an operation to save a patient's life. His reply: "I'd spend the first two minutes planning the operation." Time spent planning and organizing your priorities is time well invested.

2. Don't let anyone scramble your priorities.

You have a right to set your own agenda for success in life. Others will try to cajole you, entice you, or even bully you into setting your priorities aside so you can meet *their* priorities. They'll use guilt and manipulation to pull you away from your goals. Don't let them.

When someone asks you to take on a task, immediately decide (1) whether it is something you *choose* to do or not, and (2) what priority this task should have (if any) on your list of priorities. If you say "yes," put the task on your list in the appropriate category—Priority 1, 2, or 3—and accomplish it according to the priority it deserves. Just because someone is clamoring the loudest doesn't mean his task should be your top priority.

Keep in mind that it's okay to say, "No, I won't be able to help you." It's okay to say this without making any excuses or offering any reasons. It's okay to say, "This is my time, and I choose to spend it another way, to accomplish the goals that are important to me." You don't have to make up a lie or justify yourself. You don't owe anyone an explanation.

One of the most important time-management skills any person needs to cultivate is the skill of saying "no." Of course, you don't have to say "no" to everything. If you can afford to contribute time and energy to a worthy cause, by all means, go ahead and volunteer. But don't say "yes" just to be polite or so other people will think you're a "nice" person. Give yourself permission to politely say, "Sorry, I'm booked." Most people will respect your polite-but-firm refusal—and if they don't, that's their problem.

People will consume your time with interruptions—if you let them. They will phone you or stop by your desk and they will refuse to hang up or leave. When that happens to me, I always find it works to be polite but direct. I say, "I'm on a deadline," or, "I'm short of time right now," or, "I have to hang up now, my appendix just burst." If you want to be diplomatic about it, try saying, "I'm glad you called, let's do this again real soon," or, "I guess we've covered everything," or, "Hey, it's been great catching up with you."

And, of course, you don't have to always be at the mercy of the telephone. Let your calls be intercepted by your office receptionist, a voice mail service or an answering machine, and then pick a time convenient to you to return all the calls as a group. By grouping your return calls, you'll save even more time.

When you can, use e-mail in the place of a phone call.

People also waste your time by being late. If, for example, you have a spouse or coworker who is chronically late, you can learn ways to compensate for this person's bad habits. Allow for some wait time, and use it to relax or get work done. Keep your cellular phone or laptop computer handy or that book you've been meaning to read. Instead of fuming while you stand breathing fumes on a street corner, arrange to meet your tardy friend in a pleasant place where you won't mind cooling your heels—a favorite juice bar, art gallery, restaurant, or bookstore (I vote for the bookstore). Find creative ways to make time spent waiting productive and pleasant.

3. Understand your own motivations for wasting time—then find ways to guard against them.

There are many reasons people waste time. Some people are procrastinators, others are daydreamers. Some have a fear of failure, which results in a failure to get started, leading to a failure to finish. Some people wait for "just the right moment" or "just the right conditions." If you find yourself in one of those categories, then the only solution is to make a commitment to yourself to start right in and do first things first.

Another big psychological time-waster: obsessive perfectionism. I believe in quality and excellence as much as you do. But face it: Obsessive perfectionism does not guarantee perfection. It is possible to buff and polish a thing to the point where you spoil it. I once heard of a first-grade teacher whose classroom was adorned with the most wonderful student art. The other first-grade teachers wondered why this teacher's students produced artwork that was so much more beautiful than what their own students created. So they asked this teacher her secret. "It's simple," she said. "I've learned when to take the paper away." The same is true for us grown-ups: Sometimes "good enough" is just right; fussing over something to make it "perfect" can ruin a good thing.

Another common motivation for wasting time is *rebellion*. We revolt against the perceived intrusion of a controlling "parent," an authority figure symbolized by a boss, client, parent, clergyperson, spouse, and so forth. We play passive-aggressive games of "I'll show you!" We waste time, miss deadlines, and show up late just to prove that "Nobody can tell *me* what to do!" On some not-altogether-conscious level, we gain control over others by making them wait, by frustrating them and making them fume. In the process, we waste our own time and frustrate our own goals—but that doesn't matter as long as there is a psychological payoff, a sense of power that feeds the ego. Some people just live to generate crises. They are in constant conflict with authority, structure, calendars, deadlines, and rules. They waste enormous chunks of their lives on immature, adolescent defiance.

Another motivation for wasting time is that tingle of excitement that comes with living on the ragged edge of chaos. There is an addictive adrenaline rush that accompanies our last-minute scramble to meet a deadline. There's an exhilaration that some people gain from the challenge of racing every traffic light, beating the train at the crossing, and arriving with scant seconds to spare. There is also the wicked satisfaction of saying, "See, I told you we'd make it on time!" It's heady. It's stimulating. Okay, so it's *negative* stimulation—but once again, there's a psychological payoff. We are defiantly proud of our chaotic lives.

Sure, all that chaos and rushing around takes a toll on ourselves and the people around us—but it's *exciting*. It takes its greatest toll, however, when the excitement backfires, when we hit all the lights wrong, when the train beats us to the crossing, when the motorcycle cop clocks us doing eighty in a school zone, when we miss the appointment and lose the sale. My advice is to find some other way to get your thrills.

Another motivation for being late: "I'll just get one more thing done before I go...!" Some people are so intense about wringing every last nanosecond out of their working hours that they don't allow time for being punctual. So they arrive late and make others wait—a bad habit. It's inconsiderate to other people, whose time is also valuable. If you make an appointment, allow extra time and get there early. Time spent being on time is time well invested in making a good impression on others.

4. Put more time in your business life.

Personally, my commute time consists of a stroll down the hall to my home office. But I know that most people reading this book have a lot of commute time and travel time to deal with. That can be time wasted or time well spent—it all depends on you. If you commute, consider simplifying your life by moving closer to the office. If your company offers flexible schedules, select a travel time that avoids rush hour (preferably *before* rush hour—this will give you more time for yourself at the end of the day).

Air travel is another place where you can carve out some extra productivity. When I fly, I never check baggage. I only pack two carry-ons— a suit bag and my laptop computer case. Traveling light gets you through the airport in a flash. You'll sail past your fellow travelers as they wait around the baggage carousel. By the time they've retrieved their luggage (assuming it's not on another plane, winging its way to Patagonia), you'll be halfway to your hotel.

If you travel often, keep a checklist of your travel needs. I keep a checklist on my computer's hard drive and modify it for each trip (depending on whether I'm headed for Nome or Key West). When I pack, I have that checklist handy and never forget a thing. I also keep a kit of travel essentials in my suit bag to reduce the amount of remembering, packing, and unpacking I have to do for each trip.

> "*But* face it: Obsessive perfectionism does not guarantee perfection. It is possible to buff and polish a thing to the point where you spoil it."

The biggest time wasters for most business people are business meetings. I have endured meetings as a hapless participant—and I have chaired more than a few as well. Here are a few principles to observe when you run a meeting:

Every meeting should have a clear objective or goal that justifies its existence. Meetings should never be held purely out of habit. The agenda must be focused on a question that needs to be answered or a problem that needs to be solved. By the end of the meeting, that question or problem should have a definitive answer. If certain people are expected to give a presentation, they should be clear about these expectations (including specific objectives and time limits) at least a couple weeks before the meeting. Every meeting should end with a summation that expresses what has been accomplished and what actions are required from each participant to implement the decisions that have been reached. The meeting should have a specified time limit, and should *end on time.*

5. Put more time into your family life.

I consider family time the most valuable time in my day. I enjoy spending time talking to my wife and kids, and I don't want that precious time to be wasted on things that do not bring our family closer together. There are a number of obvious things we can do to conserve family time:

Limit the length of phone conversations (that includes everybody, kids and adults). Simplify meal preparation. Streamline meal cleanups.

Another key to conserving family time is to enlist kids in doing their part around the house, handling household chores. Household chores teach children responsibility while freeing you up to do other things. My friend Pat Williams is a father to nineteen children—four by birth, one by remarriage, and fourteen by international adoption (from such places as Romania, Brazil, and the Philippines). So he knows something about raising kids.

Pat once told me, "Our kids are expected to keep their rooms neat, put their laundry away, keep their bathrooms picked up, and take care of their own clothes and sports equipment. Our kids are no different from any others. They cut corners and sweep dirt under the carpet when they can get away with it. Don't get me wrong, they're great kids and they have good attitudes—most of the time. But kids are kids, and they'll slack off if you let them. There are times I say to myself, 'It would be simpler to just wipe that counter myself,' but if you let it slide once, it'll only get worse the next time. If you're consistent, eventually kids get to a point where they do a consistent job. That eases the strain on the whole family and gives you more time for family togetherness."

Another major time waster in most families is the television set. We rarely watch TV in our house. Sure, we have a TV and a VCR, and we use them—but sparingly. The TV is *never* on during mealtimes (except on Super Bowl Sunday!). At mealtimes, the whole family is together around the table, and we *talk*. Maybe our family is weird, but even my kids don't care for TV that much. They don't have TVs in their rooms. They don't seem to need or want to watch much television. Why? Maybe it's because my kids have a *life*.

6. Follow the Grab 15 Principle.

I saved this principle for last because it's the most important of all. I learned this principle while working on books with Bert Decker and Dru Scott Decker. Bert is the author of *You've Got to Be Believed to Be Heard* and founder of Decker Communications, Inc. His wife, Dru, is a popular business speaker and author of such books as *Customer Satisfaction*, *Stress That Motivates*, and *Women as Winners*. Dru originated the Grab 15 Principle, and Bert and Dru both promote it in their writing and speaking. It has literally *changed my life* by putting hundreds of extra hours into my working year. Here's how it works:

You've got a project you want to accomplish, but you just don't have the time. It might be that book you want to write, the exercise program you want to start, the new computer skill you want to learn, the new language you want to master. You're saving this project for that mythical "someday" when you have "more time"—which means, of course, that it will never happen.

But, thanks to Dru Scott and the Grab 15 Principle, it *can* happen. I think most of us are completely unaware of how much priceless, irreplaceable time slips through our fingers like sand through an hourglass. The Grab 15 Principle retrieves that time and uses it to make our dreams come true. Here's how it works:

First, select that project you've been wishing to accomplish.

Next, make a commitment to "grab fifteen" minutes every day without fail. Come rain or come shine, come hell or high tide, you will devote a minimum of fifteen minutes of every day to your dream. No matter how busy your day, you promise yourself that your head won't hit the pillow that night until you've done your Grab 15. Sounds too easy, right? But there are a number of good reasons why this principle is so powerful.

First reason: All those fifteen-minute snippets of time quickly add up. You might think, "What can I accomplish in fifteen minutes?" Well, let me ask you this: What could you do with an extra seventy-eight hours a year? Because even if you take Sundays off and only "Grab 15" six days a week, that works out to ninety minutes per week—*or seventy-eight hours a year.* That is time that might otherwise just fall through the cracks. You've magically added the equivalent of almost two forty-hour work weeks to your life!

Second reason: The Grab 15 Principle boosts your creativity, concentration, and retention. This is especially important if you are working on a project that requires a lot of mental focus, such as learning a language or writing a book or a play. The Grab 15 Principle keeps your head in the game. Every day, you'll spend at least fifteen minutes concentrating on your project. This provides reinforcement and continuity from day to day. Without the Grab 15 Principle, you'd be starting over from scratch every few months or years, whenever you happen to get around to your project. You'd lose tons of time just saying to yourself, "Now, where was I?" With the Grab 15 Principle, you never lose your place, never lose your momentum. Because you remain focused on your goal day after day, ideas and insights will come to you in the shower, on your commute, and while you exercise, because your project is never far from your thoughts. This makes each of your fifteen-minute sessions much more productive and effective.

Third reason: The Grab 15 Principle keeps you disciplined. It imposes a daily requirement and keeps you moving steadily toward your goal. It creates a daily habit in your life that soon becomes hard to break. If you go a day without keeping your promise to yourself, you really *miss* it—and you make sure to get back on track the next day.

Fourth and most important reason: You find it hard to stop at just fifteen minutes! You'll put in your fifteen minutes and discover you are on a roll, and you'll just keep going. That's even *more* bonus time that moves you closer to your goals.

Take it from someone who uses the Grab 15 Principle every day of his life: This is an idea that *works*.

All the time in the world

We all daydream about what we could do if we just had more time. I do that, and so do you. But you know what? We've got all the time in the world. No one—not a president nor a king nor Bill Gates nor Ted Turner—can buy one more minute of time than you already have in your day. The key to satisfaction and success in life is to make every second count. Don't wait until "someday" to live. Live *now*. Invest your time in the things that are most important in life. And what are those things?

Dru Scott once told me the story of her friend, Margaret. At the age of forty-two, after suffering a series of unexplained headaches, Margaret was told she only had a week to live. By the time the doctors found an advanced brain tumor, there was nothing they could do to save her.

When Dru got the news from Margaret's husband, she couldn't have been more stunned. Just a short time earlier, Margaret had seemed as healthy and vital as ever. She had a happy marriage, a rewarding career, two fine sons, and everything to live for. Why did she have to die? And why so cruelly and suddenly?

Two days before Margaret's death, Dru talked to her on the phone. Though the pain medication slowed and halted Margaret's speech, it could not quench her spirit. "For some reason, during these past six months,"

Margaret told Dru, "I've been thinking a lot about how I spend my time. I always thought of myself as career-oriented, but lately I've realized that my family is the most important thing in my life. These past few months, even though I had no idea I was about to die, I've spent much more time with David and the boys."

When Margaret said that, Dru flashed on her last visit in Margaret's home. She recalled Margaret gesturing toward a messy desk in one corner of the room. "I should feel guilty about that mess," Margaret had said, laughing, "but there are a lot of things more important than a clean desk. Lately, I've been concentrating on more important things—on my husband and my boys, on building family memories."

As their last conversation came to a close, Margaret said one thing that would stick in Dru's mind for the rest of her life. "It's so much easier to face what I am facing now," said Margaret, "because I've spent my time doing what really counts."

What about you and me? Are we spending our time doing what really counts? Are we investing every minute that has been given to us? Or are we just "killing time"? My friend, you have all the time in the world. Take it, invest it, and use the gift of each moment for what really counts.

5

How Do I Stop Worrying?

Bob Griese is a guy who seems incapable of worry. In fact, the very concept of worry seems alien to him, almost as if he doesn't know the meaning of the word.

When we met to work together on his book, *Undefeated*, I asked him if his first wife, Judi (who died of cancer in 1988), worried about him getting hurt when he was quarterback of the Miami Dolphins. Looking puzzled, Bob leaned back in his chair and shrugged. "Worried?" he said. "I dunno. I don't think so. Of course, I was down on the field and she was up in the stands, so I wouldn't really know. But I don't think she ever worried about me."

Later that day, I sat down with Bob and his three grown sons, Brian, Scott, and Jeff. Brian, who is now starting quarterback for the Denver Broncos, was too young to remember much of Bob's years with the Dolphins, but the older two sons, Scott and Jeff, offered some recollections of those days. At one point, Scott, the eldest, turned to Bob and said, "I remember watching your road games on TV with Mom. It drove her crazy. She worried about you all the time. She was always afraid you were going to get hurt."

"She was?" said Bob. There was that same look of puzzlement I had seen earlier in the day. It was as if he honestly couldn't understand why Judi would worry about him just because a herd of three hundred-pound defensive linemen were jumping on top of him, trying to break his bones. "She never said so."

"Well, of course, she wouldn't," said Scott.

"She used to chew on ice all the time during the games," added Jeff, "because she was so nervous."

"Really?" asked Bob.

"Oh, yeah. She had this whole big thing of ice, and she used to chew on it to relieve the tension."

Scott nodded. "And if she saw you getting into trouble on the field, she'd stand up and yell, 'Throw the ball! Get rid of it!' She knew that if you dumped the ball off, they'd go chase the guy with the ball."

Bob hadn't heard any of this before. It had never even entered his mind. "You mean she was yelling at the TV?"

"Oh, screaming!" said Scott.

"Yeah, screaming," added Jeff. "I couldn't be in the same room with her."

Bob, with the puzzled look again, "I never knew that."

"She was just as tense at the home games," added Jeff, "but she wouldn't get up and yell in the stands. She just sat there and endured it."

Scott nodded. "She *always* worried about you."

"Huh," said Bob. "I never knew that."

See what I mean? Worry is just not a part of Bob Griese's vocabulary. He also told me about the time he got his leg broken by a couple of San Diego Chargers linemen in 1972. After the play, he sat up and saw that the lower part of his leg was turned out at an odd angle. "My initial reaction," he said, "was, *Oh, geez, there goes my season.* But no use crying over it—once it's done, it's done."

"Did you worry that your career was over?" I asked.

He shrugged. "I thought, *Maybe I'll play again and maybe I won't. If it's over, well, it was fun while it lasted.* All I wanted was to get well enough to run around the yard with my boys and get out on the golf course and hit some balls. Football had been good to me, but if it was over, I could live with that."

Later, as we discussed his philosophy of life and football, Bob told me, "You can't play football all worried and tense—and you can't live your life that way. You can't be worrying that someone's gonna knock your head off. You have to say, 'I don't care if someone's gonna knock my head off—I'm gonna play my game.' I'm not saying you take stupid chances. But winning has to be more important than not getting hurt. If you don't want to get hurt, don't play the game."

And, of course, Bob is exactly right. Worry is often our biggest enemy. Worry keeps us from taking risks that bring rewards in life. Worry robs us of the joy of living. Worry can even paralyze us.

A world of worries

A recent *USA Weekend* poll showed that America is a nation of worriers. Four in ten worry about walking in their neighborhoods at night (more than half of all women, and one in five men). Since the Oklahoma City and World Trade Center bombings, one in five Americans now worries about being in a public place when a terrorist bomb goes off. Nine out of ten adults polled say the world is a more dangerous place today than when they were growing up.

> "*W*orry is often our biggest enemy. Worry keeps us from taking risks that bring rewards in life. Worry robs us of the joy of living. Worry can even paralyze us."

In the *USA Weekend* story, writer Gavin De Becker observes, "I was saddened—though not surprised—to see that fully 90 percent of Americans don't feel safer today than they did growing up." He then took a closer look at the supposedly "safer" good ol' days of the 1950s and '60s. In those days, there were no air bags, automated 911 systems, antismoking campaigns, early detection of cancer, ultrasound, organ transplants, or coronary bypass surgeries. Sure, crime rates were lower then and there was no AIDS—but there was still polio and the superpowers were planning nuclear doomsday strategies (and nearly unleashed them during the Cuban Missile Crisis). In my own memories, the '50s and '60s *seem* like a safer era simply because I was a carefree kid at the time. But when I compare then versus now through objective adult eyes, I have to admit that there is far less to worry about today than when I was a child.

But that won't keep us from worrying. According to the *USA Weekend* poll, our top worries include: (1) Being in a car crash: 54 percent. (2) Cancer: 53 percent. (3) Insufficient Social Security at retirement: 50 percent. (4) Insufficient savings for retirement: 49 percent. (5) Getting sick from tainted meat: 36 percent. (6) Alzheimer's disease: 35 percent. (7) Eating food contaminated by pesticides: 34 percent. (8) Being victimized by a violent crime: 33 percent. (9) Being unable to pay off current debts: 32 percent. (10) Being exposed to a foreign virus: 30 percent. (11) AIDS: 28 percent. (12) Being killed or injured in a natural disaster: 25 percent. Other worries that trailed in the list included loss of employment, a stock market crash, a plane crash, an IRS audit, and illness due to electromagnetic fields.[1]

What we worry about has a lot to do with where we are in life. A college student's foremost worries tend to focus on academic performance, a mother will probably worry most about the safety of her children, and an elderly person will likely worry most about financial security and health issues. Though most of us have at least some measure of worry about political, global, and environmental issues, most of our worries tend to be more focused on what could happen to *us* and our families than on what is going on in the world.

Some of the things we worry about are, in my frank opinion, rather absurd. For example, a survey in *Men's Health* magazine revealed that half of all men worry about going bald.[2] I don't doubt that statistic for a moment.

Once, when I was flying from Dallas to L.A., I was sitting in my seat, reading. A fortyish man with a full, thick head of hair came swaying down the aisle with a drink in his hand and sat down in the empty seat next to me. From his demeanor, I judged that he was on his third or fourth helping of C_2H_5OH. "Mind if I ask you a question?" he asked.

"Not at all," I said, setting my book aside.

"Does it bother you, being bald?" he asked. Blunt though it was, his observation was quite correct. I do have enough forehead for four heads.

"No," I candidly replied. "I started going bald in my twenties, and I never worried about it. I consider it a mark of distinction."

"Really!" he said. His tone suggested that he wondered why I didn't wear a bag over my head. "Well, look at this—do you think I'm going bald?" He tilted his head forward, so that I could see the top of his head. Nowhere could I see even the tiniest glimmer of scalp. This guy was *not* going bald.

"I can't see that you have anything to worry about," I said. "But I'll tell you this: I've never tried to comb my hair over the top of my head. I've never even considered hair transplants or a rug. I say if you're gonna have a head like a Crenshaw melon, then be a man and wear it proudly. If it's good enough for Michael Jordan, it's good enough for me."

He looked at me as if I had two heads—both of them bald—then he shrugged and weaved his way back to his own seat. I thought, *If he ever goes bald, it'll be from spending too much time worrying about going bald.* Many, if not most, of the things we worry about are every bit as ridiculous as the worries of my mildly inebriated friend.

A little worry is a good thing

Is there such a thing as *healthy* worry? Absolutely.

A number of times in my life, I've gotten a hunch about a certain situation. I'd get a vague tingling within, like that cliché from the *Star Wars* films: *I've got a bad feeling about this!* Sometimes I've listened to that hunch, and I've been glad I did. Other times, I've said to myself, *All the rational evidence tells me everything's okay. Forget the dumb premonition, just go with the facts.* To my regret, I sometimes discovered I should have heeded the hunch. Though not always reliable, intuition can often be a form of healthy worrying, alerting us to potential dangers and problems in our lives.

Sometimes it pays to worry about your life and health. A little sensible worry can make you more prone to buckling your seat belt, driving safely, exercising, eating right, and having regular health exams. For example, women who worry about the possibility of cervical cancer are more likely to get regular Pap smears. During the late 1980s and early '90s, there was a major campaign to alert women to the danger of cervical cancer. The result was that millions of women became more worried about their health, they went to their doctors, and cases of cervical cancer were detected early—and deaths due to this disease *fell by over 40 percent* in all age groups.[3]

So, even though most of us worry more than we should, a certain amount of worry is good for us—*if* we heed our worries and act on them. This form of worry is part of our survival instinct. It reflects our human ability to consider the future, to envision harmful scenarios, and to mentally rehearse ways of avoiding the harm.

Here's a healthy three-step way to deal with worry when a threatening problem confronts you.

Step One: Consider ways of responding to that problem.

Step Two: If there is an action that you can take to safeguard against the problem or threat, do so.

Step Three: If nothing can be done about the problem or threat, shrug, forget about it, and get on with your life.

When we brood endlessly about potential threats, imagining only the worst possible outcomes—that's when worry becomes a harmful obsession. In most cases, the worry itself is far more harmful than the thing we are worrying about. Most of the frightful outcomes we imagine never come to pass. But the process of worrying about them produces emotional stress, hypertension, heart disease, ulcers, weight gain or loss, headaches, insomnia, muscle tension, and other physical illnesses. Excessive worry is also linked to serious mental and emotional disorders, including anxiety disorder, depression, obsessive-compulsive disorder, and panic attacks.

Studies show that excessive worry upsets the balance of neurochemicals in our brains, either inhibiting or overstimulating the production of adrenaline (a stress hormone that stimulates heart action and blood pressure), gamma aminobutyric acid (a neurotransmitter that regulates brain activity), endorphins and serotonin (substances that help manage our emotions), and more. These neurochemical imbalances can cause heart palpitations, dizziness, and other symptoms.

Excessive worry can also trigger a vague sense of doom or impending death. Early in my writing career, when my financial worries were great, I often experienced a general sense of doom and thoughts of death. When times were good, these gloomy thoughts evaporated. Looking back, I realize that, on some unconscious level, my mind probably interpreted my financial worries as a threat to my mortal existence. By understanding where such thoughts come from, we begin to resolve them.

Neuroscientists have found that worry triggers intense activity in the emotional centers of the brain, disrupting the rational functioning of the "thinking brain," the cerebral cortex. In other words, worry interferes with logical, productive thinking. Worry has also been shown to impair memory and other important brain functions. That is one reason employees are generally more productive in a positive work environment than around a volatile boss and excessive pressure and stress.[4]

The net-net: Kicking the worry habit can (1) add years to your life, (2) improve your enjoyment of life, and (3) make you more productive, more successful, and a better thinker.

The profile of a chronic worrier

Everybody worries from time to time—but some people worry to a point where it hinders their effectiveness in life, and even damages their health. How do you know if you are a chronic worrier? Here are a few tests you can apply to yourself:

1. Do you find it difficult or impossible to control your worrying? Chronic worriers tend to get stuck in a cycle of worrying. They find it difficult to either let go of their worries or to take action to resolve their worries. Their worrying takes the form of an obsession that blocks positive action and change. Even when they know their worries are unfounded or exaggerated, chronic worriers feel powerless to control their worrying.

2. Do you tend to imagine the worst, most extreme outcomes of your worries? Chronic worriers tend to "awfulize" their worries. Example: The average person might worry about making a mistake on the first day of a new job, afraid of looking foolish or disappointing the new boss. But a chronic worrier might think, "If I make a mistake, I could get fired my first day on the job! I might never get another job after that. I'll lose my house, my spouse, and my kids. I'll be roaming the streets, eating out of garbage cans, and I'll probably freeze to death—all from one mistake!"

3. Do you worry even when things are going well? Chronic worriers have such a negative outlook that they think, *Life is so good, something bad has GOT to happen.* They have a morbid outlook that says, *I don't deserve to have good things happen to me.* For every silver lining, they find a thundercloud.

4. Do you strongly doubt your ability to solve a problem or manage a crisis? Chronic worriers usually lack self-confidence. They underestimate their ability to respond to crises and problems. Self-doubt often produces paralysis in an emergency. So instead of acting promptly and decisively to head off or solve the problem, chronic worriers fret and stew as their problems engulf them.

5. Were you trained as a child to be a worrier? Many chronic worriers were raised by overprotective parents who instilled a fearful, pessimistic worldview into them. Raised in a cocoon of smothering love, never allowed to risk a skinned knee or broken heart, they grew up seeing the world as hostile and threatening. So they avoid relationships, risks, and challenges. They live in a perpetual state of fear and worry.

6. Have you suffered a traumatic experience that changed your outlook on life? Many people begin life as carefree optimists, then experience a physical or emotional trauma that colors their whole outlook on life. A bride left at the altar may develop a distrust of men and romantic relationships. A plane crash survivor may be unable to board another plane. Traumatic experiences can turn anyone into a worrying pessimist.

7. Do other people comment on what a worrier you are? If others see you that way, there is probably something to it.

8. Does worry interfere with your work? Chronic worriers often pass up opportunities because they worry about taking risks or making changes. Paralyzed by worry and uncertainty, they fail to make decisions that lead to success. Their ability to focus and think logically is impaired by worry, resulting in mistakes and errors in judgment. Their constant fretting and indecision is annoying and upsetting to superiors and co-workers.

9. Does worry interfere with important relationships? The partners and friends of a chronic worrier typically complain of feeling emotionally drained, frustrated, and impatient around the worrier. The children of a chronic worrier often rebel against the worrier's overprotection and smothering affection.

10. Does worry sometimes lead to physical symptoms? Symptoms may include rapid breathing or shortness of breath, rapid or irregular heartbeat, trembling, sweating, dizziness, or insomnia. Chronic worrying can be hazardous to your health—and that's just one more thing to worry about!

It is not uncommon for an average, emotionally healthy person to read through such a list and think, *Well, that one kind of applies to me— and so does that one. Maybe I do have a problem!* Everybody worries to some degree, but that doesn't mean that you necessarily worry to an *unhealthy* degree. So if you see yourself in only two or three of the above descriptions, don't worry about it. :-)

But if you see yourself described in, say, *five or more* of the above questions, then worrying may have an unhealthy place in your life. The more completely you fit the above profile, the greater your problem is likely to be. You may even have a problem, such as clinical anxiety, that would respond well to professional therapy. If you find that you tend to worry more days than not (especially if periods of worry last a month or more); if worry hinders your sleep, your relationships, and your ability to think; or if worry has begun to affect your physical health, please seek professional help.

Strategies for winning over worry

Let's be clear about one thing: I don't claim to be an expert on psychology. As *Star Trek's* Dr. McCoy would no doubt tell me, "Dammit, Jim, you're a writer, not a doctor!" That's true, so what I offer here are not Ph.D.-level insights, but merely a few commonsense observations by someone who has had a little experience with worry. (After all, who's more qualified to talk about worry than someone who's lived the perilous life of a freelance writer?) Here, then, are some principles I've learned for overcoming worry and living a happier, more confident life:

1. Set aside a regular time for worrying. I once worked on a book with a psychiatrist in the Dallas area. He told me that this technique proved helpful for many of his worry-prone clients. You simply set aside a certain period of time—say, fifteen minutes in the morning and fifteen minutes in the evening, where you do nothing but sit and worry in a concentrated way. Sometimes, having a notebook handy and writing down your worries is a helpful part of this process. That way, you get all your worrying done and over with, you come up with solutions and ideas for resolving those worries, and then you are free to get on with the rest of your day. If you catch yourself worrying about something during the day, either dismiss it and turn your thoughts to more productive matters (work, relationships, exercise) or make a note to yourself to worry about it during your next "worry session."

2. Become informed. If you have a financial worry, sit down with your bank statement, your credit card bills, and other documents and find out exactly where you stand. If you have a health worry, go to the doctor and find out what's causing your symptoms. If you are worried about a relationship, go to that person and find out if there is or is not a problem between you. Our worries are usually out of proportion or mistaken. By becoming informed, we can usually shrink that worry down to size.

3. Talk out your worries with a trusted friend. Make sure this is a person who can keep a confidence. Talking out your worries serves several functions. Verbally expressing your worries helps to organize and clarify your thinking. Often, just talking out your worries enables you to find a solution. It also enables you to gather useful ideas and insights for resolving your worries.

4. Mobilize yourself. Instead of fretting over your worries, take action to resolve them. Be proactive. Instead of lying in bed worrying, get out of bed, take a pad and a pen and start writing down your problems and potential solutions. Make a "to do list" that prioritizes the action you must take to resolve your worries. As you take action, you will feel more confident and in control of your life—and that will put an end to your worrying.

5. Take care of your health. Good nutrition, exercise, and the appropriate amount of rest will help you feel better. The better you feel, the less worrying you are likely to do.

6. Meditate or pray. If you believe in God, commit your worries to God through meditation and prayer. You can't control all the circumstances in your life, but if you are a person of religious faith, then you certainly believe that there is a Power that oversees your circumstances. So *trust* that power. At the same time, be aware that prayer and meditation provide tangible benefits for our physical and mental health. Studies have shown that the calming disciplines of prayer and meditation trigger the release of endorphins—hormones that produce a soothing, relaxing response that enables us to control our tendency to worry.

7. Watch what you say to yourself. Psychologists call this "self-talk." Some people continually tell themselves, "I'm not smart. I'm not capable. I don't deserve anything good in life. I'm a bad person." That kind of negative thinking leads to paralysis of the will—and to worry. People do not waste time fretting and stewing in their worries when they continually say to themselves, "I can handle whatever happens. I am capable. I know how to solve problems." So be careful what you say to yourself.

8. Don't dwell on negative input (such as TV news). If you see a plane crash on TV shortly before boarding a plane, you can expect to feel more worried that your own plane may crash. If you see news coverage of home robberies or car-jackings, you will worry more about random violence. You may think it's important to be informed of such things; if so, then a higher level of worry is the price you will have to pay for being informed.

Personally, I don't think images of violence, accidents, disasters, and wars enhance my life very much. And the content of TV news is so brief and superficial that it adds little of value to my understanding of world events.

Even worse, TV news is carefully designed to provoke worry. Teasers for TV news shows are typically sensationalized scare headlines: "Is your pillow giving you brain cancer? What you don't know could kill you!" Or, "Woman injured by exploding toothpaste—could you be next?" (And in case you're getting anxious, those are made-up examples; as far as I know, pillows and toothpaste are still safe to use.) The people in TV newsrooms know: If you worry, you watch. So it's their *job* to make you worry. Turn off the news and you'll worry less—it's as simple as that.

Life is too good, and filled with too many good things to enjoy, to waste even a moment on fretting and worrying. After all, ninety-nine percent of the things we worry about never happen. And the other one percent? Well, when it happens, I'm sure you'll handle it just fine.

Questioning Relationships

6

What is Love?

When I first met supermodel Kim Alexis to work with her on her book, she told me how she met the love of her life, Ron Duguay, former forward with the New York Rangers hockey team. "My first marriage was ending," she said. "I took my kids and moved from Florida to an apartment I maintained in New York. I began house-hunting, using a real estate agent recommended by my friend, Carol Alt. She was married to Ron Greschner, the hockey player, and Carol recommended I use the real estate agent who handled most of the transactions for the Rangers' players. So I met with the agent and told her I wanted to rent a house in Connecticut. It happened that she was selling a house owned by Ron Duguay.

"I guess the agent sort of wanted to play matchmaker. So she told me about Ron and she told Ron about me. As it happened, Ron was appearing in an ad at the time, and the ad agency needed a female model to appear in the ad with him. Recalling what the real estate agent had said about me, he asked, 'How about Kim Alexis?' He thought it would be a great way to meet me. The advertising people said, 'Sure—if we can get her.' So they contacted me and I took the job.

"I took my boys and our nanny to the location for the shoot. At one point, I was busy working with the photographer. I assumed the nanny was watching the boys, but she was talking to somebody, not paying attention. Just then, one of my boys wandered over by a fountain, and Ron followed my son to make sure he wouldn't fall in. When I looked and saw Ron looking after my son, I was so impressed. From then on, I just wanted to touch him—to touch his hand, his face, his back. I think it was his strength combined with his gentleness that won my heart."

About fifteen months later, Kim and Ron were married, and they are happy together to this day. They've found something the whole world is looking for—the answer to one of the deepest questions of the human heart:

What is love?

One word for four loves

There are a number of distinct kinds of love. Unfortunately, the English language has only one word to describe them all. The ancient Greeks, from Aristotle to the writers of the Greek New Testament, had four different words for four different kinds of love. The first love most of us come to know is the love between a parent and child. The Greeks called this *storge* (pronounced STORE-gay), an affection between unequals. This term was also used to describe the unequal but affectionate relationship between a mentor and his student or even between a human master and a pet dog.

Storge-affection is a form of love in which one side (the child) has needs and the other side (the parent) meets those needs. It is a complementary love relationship in which both sides find fulfillment. The parent embraces and cares for the child, and the child clings to the parent for comfort and security. Each feels *storge*-affection for the other.

The next love most of us come to know is what the Greeks called *philia* or friendship love. This love is also called "brotherly love," which is where Philadelphia, "the City of Brotherly Love," gets its name. *Philia* is a love of between equals. In its broadest sense, it is a love for all humankind—a sense of responsibility for the welfare of your neighbor. But it is more particularly a love for a friend. We discover *philia*-love early in life, as soon as we begin to make friends, as soon as we find one or two people we enjoy being with and doing things with. We discover *philia*-love in the sandbox or the tree house of childhood, and we rediscover the warmth and pleasure of *philia*-love again and again as we grow older. Some of us are fortunate enough to make *philia-love* friendships that last a lifetime.

The third form of love that the Greeks spoke of (and the *first* form most of us think of when we hear the word "love") is *eros*. We tend to associate the word *eros* with sexual or romantic love. But in the original Greek language, *eros* had a broader meaning than that. *Eros* is also a love of beauty, art, and nature. In that sense, it is *eros* you feel when you admire a piece of Limoges china, a beautiful painting, a haunting sonata, or a mint-condition Mickey Mantle rookie card. You admire it, you want it, you wish to possess it. Erotic love says, "I love you, I need you, I want you."

Eros-love between two people begins with the thrilling experience called "falling in love"—that is, attraction and infatuation. It's one of the most exciting and emotionally intense experiences of the human condition. Some couples expect that kind of intensity to last forever. That, of course, is not realistic. What makes this experience so intense is that it is *new*. It's an adventure of exploring and discovering another person. Once that person becomes more familiar, with all his or her flaws and faults, the newness and the intensity are bound to recede.

What happens when the passion of eros begins to lose its intensity? People often panic and think, *Oh, no! I'm falling out of love! I need to go find someone else to fall in love with so I can get a new thrill!* Others, however, manage to build a warm and satisfying relationship that stands the test of time. How do they do it? How do you make the love you feel for another last?

"Falling in love" is as easy as falling off a log, but *living* in love seems as hard as walking a tightrope. You'll recall that I mentioned four kinds of love that the ancient Greeks spoke of. So far, we have only discussed three. It is this fourth kind of love that enables us to walk that tightrope and truly live in love. What is the name of that fourth kind of love? It is called *agape*. The word looks as if it refers to one's mouth hanging ajar, but this Greek word is actually pronounced ah-GAW-pay.

What does *agape* have that *eros* and the other loves do not? Answer: *Agape lasts.*

A love between unequals

Bear with me and I will tell you what *agape*-love is and how you can find it. But first, it's important to see how these various forms of love combine together—because the *harmonizing* of these different forms of love is the key to building a love that lasts. We have already seen that *eros*-love cannot endure by itself—that's the bad news. Fortunately, however, *eros* easily combines with other forms of love. Some of these combinations result in rich, lasting relationships (though others, unfortunately, produce unhealthy, ill-matched relationships). Let's take a closer look at these combinations and see which ones work—and which do not.

First, what if we combined *eros* with *storge*? Would that be a lasting love? *Storge*, remember, is a love between unequals, like the love between parent and child. It is not uncommon to see relationships with a strong *eros-storge* component—but they are rarely healthy relationships.

One example is the man who approaches love with a "rescuer" mentality. He is drawn to "women in distress." He may rescue women by meeting their financial needs, or by taking them out of a situation with an abusive boyfriend, or by rescuing them from themselves, trying to help them get off of alcohol or drugs.

Why does this kind of man feel compelled to rescue needy women? Because he believes a needy woman will *need him*. If he rescues her, he becomes her hero. In his insecurity, he doesn't feel competent to attract a woman who is his equal, but if he can "save" her, he becomes "superior" and he feels more attractive, competent, and confident.

There are a number of reasons this is an unhealthy scenario. One problem is that many "women in distress" never get out of the distress mode. Distress is their modus operandi, their way of coping with life, their way of getting sympathy and support. Some manipulative women instinctively know that by being perpetually "helpless," they can always attract a guy who is eager to bail them out. They reward him with the magic words, "My hero!" If they enter into a long-term relationship, the "hero" may eventually tire of constantly bailing her out. What seemed attractive to him at first will, in time, become tiresome and boring.

Another problem with this scenario is that the damsel may only be in temporary distress. Our hero may be the hero of the hour—but what if she later decides she no longer needs rescuing? If he continually tries to rescue her and she feels competent to handle her own life, thank you very much, then a new dynamic sets in: She resents him for being "too controlling," and he resents the fact that he is no longer needed.

And there is another *storge* + *eros* combination that is equally unhealthy. Women who like to be in control tend to marry passive men who won't challenge their control. It's a comfortable arrangement for both sides, because these men like to have a strong-willed woman who will (metaphorically) cut their steak and wipe their chins for them, make their decisions for them, and assume a quasi-parental role. It's a *storge*-love relationship between unequals.

At first it seems like a great arrangement. She likes being the boss, he's comfortable being bossed. (Sometimes, there's an added bonus for the passive guy in that he now has a bossy, controlling wife to challenge his bossy, controlling mother.) But soon the strong-willed woman discovers that the very trait that attracted her to this guy now drives her nuts. It's great that her man never challenges *her*—but the spineless little noodle won't challenge anyone else, either! He won't ask for a raise. He doesn't object when people cut in front of him at the supermarket. He has no sales resistance, no drive, no ambition. Ultimately, no woman, not even a strong-willed woman, wants to stay married to Casper Milquetoast.

The net-net: *Storge*-love and *eros*-love don't mix well, because the result is a pairing of unequals. An *eros*-love between unequals can never be a lasting, satisfying love. Authentic love must be a love between equals.

A love between equals

So if *storge*-love is not the right mixer for *eros*, what is?

Well, there is *philia*, friendship love. *Philia* is a love between equals. You probably know of many situations where a platonic friendship has blossomed into romantic love. These are often the richest, most lasting relationships because they begin not with the selfish attraction of *eros* but the selfless affection of *philia*; the *eros* is added later after an abiding friendship is already established. Friends tend to be more focused on reality than lovers, who are focused only on each other's eyes. Friends have the capacity to look into the future; lovers tend to live in an eternal present. As C.S. Lewis writes in *The Four Loves*, "We picture lovers face to face, but friends side by side; their eyes look ahead."[1] A love made up of both *philia* and *eros* is a good foundation for a genuine, lasting love.

But there is another Greek conception of love that is even more durable than *philia* or friendship love. That love, as I've already mentioned, is called *agape*. *Agape*-love is very different from *storge*, *philia*, and *eros*, because it does not take place in the emotions or the affections. *Agape* takes place in the will. *Agape* is not a feeling, it's a decision. No one can ever "fall in *agape*." *Agape*-love is a commitment to love even at those times when the one you love is not lovely or lovable.

The beauty of *agape* is that is mixes well with every other form of love. And when it mixes with another form of love, it elevates that love to the highest possible degree. Sometimes in a parent-child relationship, *storge* is not enough. Especially in the teen years, a child can become defiant and obnoxious, and it's hard to feel any *storge*-affection for such a rebellious brat. But if you make a commitment to show *agape* love to that child, you and the child will get through it.

Sometimes it's hard to feel *philia* (brotherly love) toward a friend who has let you down, or the drunk on the street who threw up on your shoes, or the neighbor who swore at you over the back fence. But when you mix *agape* with *philia*, you make a willful commitment to forgive your friend, to provide help to the drunk, and to be tolerant and understanding toward your nasty neighbor.

Agape is inclusive, not exclusive; it gives us the ability to love those we have never met. A person who knows how to *agape*-love one person can love *all* people, because all people are really the same. Skin color makes no difference. Nor does language, national origin, religion, political affiliation, or sexual orientation. We can love those with whom we vehemently disagree. Liberals can love conservatives, and vice versa. The rich can love the poor, and vice versa. Christians and Jews and Moslems can love each other.

We have already seen how mixing *agape*-love with *philia*-friendship can make a stronger, more lasting love relationship. Now, when you add *agape*-love to that foundation of *eros* and *philia*, you really have a powerful combination. There are times, over the span of a romantic relationship, when the person we love is not very lovely or lovable. At those times, *eros* alone is not enough. Feelings of *philia*-friendship can only go so far. But the rock-solid commitment of *agape*, rooted not in the feelings but in the will, enables a love-relationship to endure to the end of life itself.

Feelings change, but a commitment of the will is as durable as we *choose* to make it. Feelings of *eros* are beyond our control, but an *agape* decision is entirely within our ability to control. *Agape* love is the ultimate in unselfishness. In a romantic relationship, it is a decision to embrace everything that is important to the person we love.

Agape-love is a knowing and understanding love. It is willing to take the time to plumb the depths of another human soul. People are made up of many subtle layers. If we only care to know the outermost layer, we do not truly love. For example, if your lover becomes angry with you, you have several options. You can ignore, you can attack—or you can try to understand the deep and underlying reasons for the anger.

If you truly *agape*-love someone, you don't just blow off that person's feelings. You make the effort to grasp the soul-reality of that person. You set aside your prejudices, preconceptions, and stereotypes and you delve into that person's innermost being. To truly love is to know and understand.

Agape-love is an accepting love. It's the ability to honestly see a person as he or she is and to continue loving that person, flaws and all. It doesn't mean we don't want the people we love to ultimately grow beyond their faults and failings. It doesn't mean we ignore their character flaws and indulge their weak side. But while they are working on growth and maturity, we accept them and love them right where they are on their journey.

Ultimately, *agape*-love is a healing love. It takes all the pain and failures of our lives and reweaves them into something beautiful. In his book *Mortal Lessons*, surgeon Richard Selzer tells the story of a healing act of *agape*-love he witnessed at a patient's hospital bedside:

> I stand by the bed where a young woman lies, her face postoperative, her mouth twisted in palsy. A tiny twig of the facial nerve, the one to the muscles of her mouth, has been severed. She will be thus from now on.... To remove the tumor in her cheek, I had to cut the little nerve.
>
> Her young husband is in the room. He stands on the opposite side of the bed, and together they seem to dwell in the evening lamplight, isolated from me, private....
>
> "Will my mouth always be like this?" she asks.
>
> "Yes," I say, "it will. It's because the nerve was cut."
>
> "I like it," the husband says. "It's kind of cute." ...He bends to kiss her crooked mouth, and I am so close I can see how he twists his own lips to accommodate hers, to show her that their kiss still works.[2]

You ask what love is? *That* is your answer.

How Can I Have a Better Relationship?

When I first met Super Bowl champion Bob Griese at his home in North Carolina, I was impressed with what a great relationship Bob and his wife, Shay, seem to have. They're just so *right* for each other. I spent three days visiting and working with them, and my last day there, I asked Shay how she and Bob first met.

"We met on a flight in 1990," she explained. "I'm very outgoing and talkative, and Bob is just the opposite. He was sitting there in his window seat, hiding behind his copy of *USA Today*, and I sat down next to him and started talking—'Hi, my name is Shay! How are you? What are you reading? Do you play gin? I bet I can beat you at cards!'"

Shay didn't know that Bob Griese was an ABC sportscaster and former Miami Dolphins quarterback. "All I knew," she said, "was that I would be sitting next to this guy for a couple of hours, and I didn't think we should sit there like strangers on an elevator. So I tried to get him to open up—but he wouldn't talk! Everything I said, he'd answer in words of one syllable, and he'd raise his paper a little higher.

"Finally, I talked him into a game of cards. He sat in a window seat, and I could see all his cards reflected in the window—so I won every hand! Maybe that's what won him over. Bob is so competitive, he just hates to lose—yet he couldn't beat me!"

At that time, Bob Griese had been widowed for two years and was raising Brian, the youngest of his three sons, alone. Shay and Bob became friends. "For the next few months," Shay told me, "we'd call each other every once in a while, or maybe have lunch. It wasn't a romantic thing—just friends. Brian was still at home, and Bob was totally focused on being a full-time dad. I thought that was great—I admired Bob's devotion to his boys."

Bob and Shay were married in 1994, four and a half years after they met. Bob told me, "Shay has been incredibly good for me and the boys. She's been very kind to my sons, and they know she's been good for me. They're glad she's keeping an eye on their old man." When you meet people who are just *right* together, you know it, you see it in the way they relate to each other. Bob and Shay Griese are a couple like that.

How do you find a great relationship like that? Is it luck? Is it magic? Or is it a matter of maturity, character, and hard work?

How do people come together?

The place to begin is where all romantic relationships begin—the point where two people meet, are attracted to each other, and grow to love each other. You may be thinking, *But I'm already in a relationship. I don't need dating advice. I need to know how to make my relationship work better.* Fact is, knowing how the two of you first became a couple can shed a lot of light on the issues you are dealing with now. And if you do happen to be in the beginning stages of a relationship, you're just in time!

One of the great mysteries of relationships is the mystery of attraction, of how two people come together. Dr. Harville Hendrix, founder of the Institute for Relationship Therapy, observes in *Getting the Love You Want* that attraction is rooted in biology. Both men and women follow mating patterns that favor the survival of the human species. Men are drawn to youth, beauty, and a voluptuous figure because these attributes indicate a prime candidate for childbearing. This is not to say that the guy with the smooth pick-up lines is consciously looking for someone to be the mother of his children. On a conscious level, he may be looking for nothing more than a roll in the hay. But eons of evolutionary forces have formed his taste in women with a goal of encouraging sex to take place. The sex act tends to produce children, and children ensure the survival of the species.

And what do women want? Well, most women *say* they want a guy who is tender and compassionate, a guy who is content to spend hours just cuddling. But there is often a disparity between what we consciously *think* we want and what we are unconsciously attracted to. So what kind of guys do women *really* go for? According to Hendrix, it is the *homo sapiens* version of the alpha-ape. (Which may explain why so many women who *say* they want Mr. Tender-and-Compassionate end up with a knuckle-dragging Neanderthal.) In less civilized times, it was the domineering, aggressive male who brought the largest share of the kill back to the cave and best ensured the survival of the family group.

Romantic attraction is like an iceberg: Only 10 percent of the process meets the eye; the other 90 percent lurks beneath the surface of our conscious awareness. That's why this issue is so complex and mysterious. Hendrix identifies two primary ways the primitive, unconscious parts of our brains (the parts most closely associated with mating and sex) cause us to be attracted to certain people, often with devastating results.

1. Reconstructing childhood situations

Romantic attraction has a lot to do with the fact that people are unconsciously driven to symbolically reconstruct the dynamics that existed with their childhood caregivers. "No matter what their conscious intentions," writes Hendrix, "most people are attracted to mates who have their caretakers' positive *and* negative traits, and, typically, the negative traits are more influential."[1]

Why would we unconsciously seek out people who have the *negative* traits of our parents or other childhood caregivers? There are a number of possible answers. For one, we tend to seek what is familiar, even if the familiar is also painful and dysfunctional. For another, the primitive part of ourselves is attempting to reconstruct the childhood situation so that old, unresolved childhood conflicts can be replayed in the present. Unfortunately, these old conflicts cannot be won.

A few years ago, I worked with psychologist Jim Osterhaus on his book, *Questions Couples Ask Behind Closed Doors*. During our discussions, he explained the mystery of attraction this way: "The primitive part of our brain continually tries to heal the wounds of childhood, resolve childhood conflicts, and compensate for the emotional deficits of childhood. It confuses the image of the parent with the image of the potential mate and says, in effect, 'Here is someone like Mom or Dad. If I marry this person, I can carry on the struggle I began in childhood—a struggle for love and acceptance. If I win this time, I can have everything that was denied me in childhood: security, affirmation, and love.'

"This is why children of alcoholic parents marry alcoholic spouses with numbing regularity. It's why children of abusive parents find themselves paired with abusive spouses with amazing frequency. Children of unloving parents marry emotionless, uncaring mates again and again. The primitive brain compels us toward those who unconsciously remind us of our parents."

Consciously, we may only be aware of the positive traits of the other person—but the primitive part of our brains is attracted by both the positive *and negative* traits. Once the primitive brain is satisfied that the original situation, with all its familiar struggles, has been restored, the primitive brain rejoices: *The idealized mate has been found!* Feelings of attraction ensue.

Harville Hendrix has a word for the idealized mate: The *imago* (from the Latin word for "image"). It is a template imprinted on our primitive brains. Whenever we meet someone who is a prospective partner, the primitive brain compares that person with the template or imago of the idealized mate. "Unconsciously," says Hendrix, "you have compared every man or woman that you have met to your imago. When you identified a close match, you felt a sudden surge of interest."[2]

When we find a person who closely matches our imago, our idealized mate, we often experience several intense feelings: *recognition* ("I feel as if I already know you"), *reunification* ("Being with you feels like I'm home at last"), *timelessness* ("It's like I've always known you"), and *necessity* ("I can't live without you"). Hendrix notes that all of these feelings are rooted in the fact that our imago is composed largely of the image of our caretakers. So it's hardly surprising that there are feelings of recognition and reunification: finding someone who matches our childhood caretakers makes us feel we have returned home. It's not surprising we have a feeling of timelessness, for we can't recall a time when we didn't know our childhood caretakers. Nor is the feeling of necessity, of "I can't live without you," surprising; when we were children, that sense of life-and-death dependency was literally true.

2. The missing aspects of the self

The second major factor in attraction, notes Hendrix, is *the missing or repressed aspects of ourselves*. We all grow up feeling criticized for negative traits. We are told we are too boisterous—or too quiet. We are too dependent—or too much of a loner. We are too fat—or too skinny. We are too impulsive—or too hesitant. Over time, we repress aspects of ourselves in order to be accepted by others. We disown and deny the parts of ourselves we cannot face. Then we walk around feeling like a jigsaw puzzle with major pieces missing.

Along comes someone who seems to possess the repressed, denied, and missing parts of ourselves. When we are around that person, we don't feel incomplete anymore. We feel *whole*. In fact, many people describe their romantic relationship by saying, "He/she makes me feel complete." Sounds good—but is it healthy? In many cases, no. The relationship may well be based on a faulty premise and unhealthy expectations: "This is the person who will meet all my needs and fill up everything I lack. In fact, I must have this person completely and all the time or I am incomplete."

Such relationships often become emotional sinkholes, riddled with unhealthy obsession and possessiveness. The two partners seem to merge into one. At first, all the clinging and emotional fusion is exciting and ecstatic—but one partner often wakes up to find himself or herself in a smothering relationship, unable to breathe.

But those are extreme cases. Fact is, being attracted to someone with qualities we lack is perfectly healthy as long as we don't take it to the point of extreme obsession. There are good, healthy reasons why opposites attract. My wife and I, for example, have a number of opposing traits that sometimes complement each other—and sometimes conflict with each other. On the whole, we build on the complementary nature of our personalities and abilities. When you can do that, you have the makings of a great partnership, because there is a healthy division of labor. I do what I'm good at, my wife does what she's good at, and between the two of us it all gets done.

Building a healthy, lasting relationship

Many people today seem to approach relationships with an attitude that says, "Somewhere out there is my perfect match. When I find my soul mate, everything's going to be just right." Let's say Rachel and Ross fall in love. They either get married or move in together, thinking this is "it," this is "the perfect match."

Before long, as happens in every relationship, problems and irritations arise between Rachel and Ross. A sense of disappointment sets in—then turns to panic. "Oh, no!" Ross says to himself, "I made a mistake! All of Rachel's idiosyncrasies that I used to think were so cute are driving me up the wall!"

And Rachel, who learned all about love from romance novels, says to herself, "Oh, no! Ross isn't my perfect match, my soul mate, after all! If we were a match, everything would be perfect, we would never have fights, and he wouldn't have all those annoying habits and dumb ideas!"

So Rachel and Ross bail out of their relationship—which, of course, stuns all of their friends. After all, they seemed so right for each other. Ross explains the breakup to his friends, Chandler and Joey, saying, "We just weren't compatible." And Rachel tells her friends, Monica and Phoebe, "We just grew apart." And once again, Rachel and Ross resume their lonely quests for the mythical "perfect match."

Time for a bite of a reality sandwich. There is no "perfect match" for you anywhere on this planet. Sure, there are people who would be a good fit for your personality, temperament, life goals, and so forth—but nobody is *the* perfect fit. There are no tailor-made relationships. Every relationship is strictly an off-the-rack proposition. That means alterations must be made in order to improve the fit—alterations in the other person and alterations in *you*.

Problems, disappointments, and conflict don't mean it's time to dump the relationship or that you married the wrong person. Some people trot off to divorce court at the first sign of trouble. Their big mistake is in giving up too soon on a relationship that could have been saved with work and maturity. Very often, if people would just hang in, give more and demand less, they would ultimately reach a place of satisfaction in the relationship.

Here are five practical ways to build a happier, healthier relationship:

1. Set healthy boundaries.

I've worked with psychologist Jim Osterhaus on three books—one on marriage relationships, one on relationships with difficult parents, and one on business relationships in the workplace. In each of those three books, Jim stressed the importance of healthy boundaries in all relationships. The word "boundaries" may sound like so much psychobabble, but in my own experience I have found that healthy boundaries are a crucial dimension of a healthy relationship.

"Boundaries," Jim explains, "say that certain people, certain actions, certain intrusions are not permitted here. This is who I am, this is who you are, and this is how we should behave toward each other. Anything that falls outside of these limits is not allowed." There are two kinds of boundaries that define a healthy relationship: boundaries *around* the relationship and boundaries *within* the relationship.

First, there must be healthy boundaries *around* a couple, creating a zone of safety against intrusions from parents, siblings, and in-laws. When one partner has not "left home" by separating from parents and siblings, the relationship is bound to have big problems. This partner may spend all of his or her free time over at Mom and Dad's. Or parents and siblings may feel free to walk in on the couple unannounced, or criticize the way they live their lives, or meddle in their relationship.

> "*...Healthy boundaries are a crucial dimension of a healthy relationship.*"

Another important boundary around the relationship is the boundary between the couple and the outside world. Flirting, phone sex, and cybersex are behaviors that violate this boundary. So does acting disloyally by criticizing or embarrassing one's partner in front of other people. A person with healthy boundaries doesn't reveal secrets of the marriage relationship—sexual intimacies, shame issues, and so forth—to other people. The boundary around the couple is a zone of protection that makes intimacy possible. Without healthy boundaries, there is no trust. Without trust, there is no intimacy.

Second, there must be healthy boundaries *within* the relationship. "The paradox of a good marriage," says Jim Osterhaus, "is that two separate people can enter into a relationship so intimate that it borders on emotional fusion, yet each partner maintains his or her own individuality. Each partner must be able to say, 'This is who I am as opposed to you. These are *my* thoughts, *my* feelings, *my* desires, *my* goals.' The boundaries within a relationship safeguard the individuality of both partners."

It's okay, for example, for a couple not to do everything together. It's healthy for each partner to have his or her own interests, hobbies, clubs, friends, and activities. It's perfectly healthy for one partner to take an occasional shopping trip with friends to Carmel-by-the-Sea, or enjoy a golf weekend with buddies to Marco Island, or spend time alone at a mountain retreat for spiritual reflection. These are healthy boundaries within a relationship that serve to insure and maintain each partner's individuality.

It's possible, however, to take boundaries too far. When a couple maintains separate finances, sleeps in separate bedrooms, or routinely takes separate vacations, then the boundaries between each partner have become too rigid. Particularly in a marriage (which is a more committed relationship than living together), there should be no guardedness and wariness between two partners. Healthy boundaries require a delicate balancing act: Partners should be distinct but not separate, bonded but not bound to each other.

2. Build trust by making and keeping commitments.

Every healthy relationship is built on a foundation of trust. And trust between two people is based on the ability to make and keep a promise. One reason it is important to know a person well before entering into a committed relationship is that it takes time to build trust. Only when you have a certain depth of experience with another person do you know you can depend on that person to be faithful, responsible, and true.

People sometimes come into a relationship with a damaged capacity for trust. Some people fear being engulfed by others, so they create distance in relationships, surrounding themselves with emotional armor. Others fear abandonment, so they become clingy in relationships, and constantly require reassurance that they will not be left alone. Ironically, those who fear engulfment and those who fear abandonment often attract each other, creating a vicious cycle: One retreats from engulfment, causing the other to feel abandoned; the one who feels abandoned pursues the one who fears engulfment, causing even more frantic retreat. The only way to break the cycle is for *both* sides to learn to trust.

How do we build trust? First, both partners should make sure that any past emotional issues are brought out into the open and resolved (such as violated trust in childhood or previous romantic relationships). Professional counseling may be needed to provide insight into those problems.

Second, both partners should commit themselves to a promise. This is why marriage is qualitatively different from living together. Some people say that marriage is "just a piece of paper," but it is more than that. It is a vow, a binding promise. A promise is a declaration of our intentions and a commitment to carry out those intentions to completion. When people show that they can make and keep promises, trust just naturally ensues.

3. Practice healthy communication habits.

Communication problems in relationships take various forms. One of the most treacherous is *mind reading*. It is common for people, especially in the early stages of a relationship, to feel so fused to each other that they assume (1) they can read their partner's mind and (2) their partner can read theirs. There is a dangerous and unspoken expectation: "You should know what I want before I even ask." When the partner *doesn't* know, a new assumption sets in: "My partner knows what I want, but is *deliberately* trying to frustrate me!" These assumptions set the stage for bitter conflict.

Uncommunicated expectations are common pitfalls in relationships. Whenever we have expectations of our partner, they should be communicated clearly: "I want you to be more friendly to my parents when they come to dinner tonight." Or "I'd like you to take responsibility for cleaning the bathrooms every Saturday." We all have expectations, and one way or another, they will be expressed. If they are not expressed via clear, healthy verbal communication, they will be expressed through "the silent treatment," sarcasm, or open warfare.

Uncommunicated expectations are dangerous to a relationship, especially when it comes to sex: "If she doesn't know when I'm in the mood for sex after twenty years, then she must not care about my needs." Or "I wish he'd take sex more slowly and gently—but it's too embarrassing to talk about." But you *need* to talk about it. Lack of communication creates distrust and distance and destroys intimacy.

One of the most overlooked aspects of communication is listening. Each side needs to make a conscious effort to listen—*really listen*—to what the other side is saying. We need to listen constructively, trying to put the best spin on what the other person is saying—not the worst. We need to listen actively, repeating back in our own words what the other person said so that he or she knows we really do hear and understand. We need to listen attentively, actually hearing the other person instead of merely planning our rebuttal. Partners in a relationship must learn to communicate as partners—not as opponents.

4. Work as a team to solve conflicts.

Every couple has conflict, but conflict doesn't have to destroy a relationship. In fact, a lovingly resolved conflict can actually bring a couple closer. Loving couples know how to "fight fair" when conflict arises. They focus on restoring the relationship, not winning the fight. One of the most helpful strategies for resolving conflict in a relationship is to have a set of rules that you both agree on ahead of time—rules for "fighting fair." Here are some good ones to adopt:

- *Stay in the present.* Don't dredge up old wounds. When you bring up the past, you show your own failure to forgive.

- *Avoid lecturing.* If you have a complaint, give concrete examples, not generalizations. Instead of saying "You're such a jerk," say, "I was embarrassed when you made armpit noises in front of my mother this morning." Generalities make people feel personally attacked. Concrete examples give people specific behaviors to work on.

- *Use "I" statements instead of "you" statements.* Compare these two statements which express the same complaint:

  "You're so busy and unavailable! You're never home, and when you are home, you're always holed up with that stupid computer!"

  "I've been really lonesome lately. I miss spending time with you."

  Which statement is more likely to lead to resolution and greater intimacy?

- *Always be honest.* Honesty is not only the right thing to do, it's smart. Lies and evasions only trip you up. Use times of conflict as opportunities to exchange deep truths about yourselves. Honesty produces trust; trust leads to intimacy.

- *Avoid blaming.* When we blame, we try to make ourselves the winner and our partner the loser. A healthy relationship is not about winners and losers. It's about loving each other and restoring the relationship.

- *Fight about one thing at a time.* When issues proliferate, chaos results. So stay focused. Resolve one issue before going on to the next.

- *Don't issue ultimatums.* An ultimatum is a demand with a

threat attached. Enemies issue ultimatums to each other. Partners in a relationship treat each other with love, understanding, and respect—not threats.

- *Lay down your verbal weapons.* Never use words to hurt. The longer you know a person and the closer you become, the better you know that person's "hot buttons"—the things you can say or do that will really set your partner off. If you truly love your partner, *never* push those "hot buttons." Hurtful words, once spoken, can't be called back; they may be forgiven in time—but can they be forgotten? Use words to build up your relationship, not tear it down. "I want a divorce!" is one of the most destructive things you can say. And how about this one: "Not only that, but you're lousy in bed, too!" Even if you are eventually forgiven, don't expect a red-hot love life after a shot like that.

- *Don't give up.* Don't turn your back or walk out of the room. If the argument drags on and you need a break, then take a break. Don't insist on "talking it out right here and now" if you or your partner needs half an hour to calm down and get collected. You can mutually choose to finish the argument at a later time.

5. Persevere.

There are very few Cinderella stories in the real world of relationships, very few couples who find love at first sight and live happily ever after. In fact, most people probably reach a point (or several points) in their relationship where they ask themselves, "How did I get stuck in this relationship?" Immature people often give up on a perfectly good relationship at this stage. Mature people—people with real depth of soul—persevere and find a deeper level of love than they ever imagined. True, there are some relationships that shouldn't be saved—but a truly unsalvageable relationship usually involves *extreme* problems of abuse, alcoholism, addiction, or adultery.

I'm convinced that most broken relationships could be saved *if* both partners would make a commitment to love each other through the difficult passages of their relationship. As columnist Leonard Pitts, Jr., of the *Miami Herald* once observed, "An old friend of mine says that 90 percent of the time his marriage makes him glad he is alive. The other 10 percent it makes him want to say, 'Please kill me now.' The trick is to get through the ten by trusting the ninety. Sometimes marriage is just an act of faith."

Couples who lovingly persevere through the passages of a relationship generally reach a place of peace, security, and satisfaction with each other. Psychiatrist M. Scott Peck describes how he and his wife, Lily, went through such a passage in their relationship. They reached a point where, after twenty years of marriage, they had "negotiated boundaries and rules" that enabled them to coexist. Still, they were both "significantly depressed" over their relationship, unsure if their marriage could or even should survive. For *ten years*, from the twenty- to the thirty-year mark of their marriage, they stuck with a depressing marriage. Amazingly, at that point, a change came over their relationship. Peck explains:

> Gradually, almost without willing it, some of Lily's foibles began to amuse me. I slowly realized that each of her shortcomings was the flip side of a virtue that I very much admired and depended upon. Similarly she observed that some of the things about me she used to curse were quite natural side effects of certain gifts of mine that she herself lacked. It slowly dawned on us that we meshed rather well. We became adept at consulting each other. What once had been cause for friction and rage now became a cause for celebration—celebration of our smooth interdependence. By the thirty-year mark our previously depressing marriage was mostly fun, and now seven years later, when we are well embarked into retirement, it is a delight.[3]

This is one of the great truths of great relationships: If you persevere through the dark passages of your relationship, you will eventually emerge into the sunlight of a safe, secure love that has ripened, matured, and stood the test of time. And you'll know that it was worth it.

8

How Can I Get Past Feeling Angry?

One screaming father, his three little daughters cowering in their beds, while their mother tries to pull the dad out of the room. The father's ominous threat: "If you don't get to sleep right now—!" The door slamming hard enough to dislodge plaster from the walls. This was the scene described by newspaper writer Christopher Scanlon in an article headlined "Daddy's Rage." Most surprising of all, the Daddy in the newspaper story was Scanlon himself.

He went on to describe what he heard after slamming the door and stamping away from his daughters' room. The sniffling and whimpering of his three girls. His wife's apologetic explanation of their father's rage: "Daddy loves you very much. He's just tired, and he wants you to go to sleep....Sometimes parents get upset, and they do things they shouldn't." And he described what he felt: the pounding pulse in his temples, the ragged throat, the rising sense of remorse and self-hate over lashing out in anger—*again*.

Christopher Scanlon is not an abuser, nor a violent man. He's a father who courageously admits to a common problem: "All my life," he writes, "I have struggled with anger....At the office, I'm friendly, easy-going, generally considered a nice guy. It's only at home that I display this vein-popping, larynx-scraping rage....Why must loved ones bear the brunt of anger?"

Anger can work for you—and against you

Anger is a difficult emotion for most of us to deal with—or even acknowledge. Some of us are brought up to think of anger as "bad" or "sinful." But anger is just an emotion. While we can usually control our behavior, it is much harder to control our emotions. An emotion isn't good or bad, an emotion just *is*. Being angry may make us *feel* bad, it may be extremely unpleasant, but it is not "bad" or "wrong" to feel angry. With a few basic insights into what anger is and how it works, you *can* learn to manage your response to anger.

The emotion of anger produces powerful physiological reactions. It serves as an alarm system, alerting the body to take action against an outside threat. The emotion of anger is a survival mechanism, part of the primal "fight-or-flight" response. At one time, anger helped prepare our ancestors to either face down a bear (fight) or run from a saber-toothed tiger (flight). The problem, of course, is that while we seldom deal with bears or tigers anymore, the fight-or-flight response still works like it used to. The primitive parts of the brain are unable to distinguish between a tiger-shaped threat to our existence and an annoying but nonlethal insult from a passing motorist. Result: Even when the "threat" is nothing more than an upraised finger, we become furious and our bodies go into full-blown fight-or-flight mode.

What are the physical effects of the fight-or-flight response? First, feelings of anger activate increased levels of adrenaline and cortisol in the body. These secretions raise the blood pressure and quicken the pulse for battle. Arteries redirect blood flow to the muscles for extra clobbering power. The blood platelets become thick and gooey, so the blood will clot in case of injury. Throbbing with rage, the individual is ready for battle.

By understanding the physiological dimension of anger, we can begin to get our anger under control. For example, some people may have adrenal glands that release more fight-or-flight chemicals into the bloodstream. Result: When angry, they may feel more threatened, more tense, more defensive—and that may cause them to react in a more extreme way. It may be harder for them to maintain control than a person whose body puts out less adrenaline. If you are one of these people, it is important to recognize this fact and avoid putting yourself into situations that may trigger your body's fight-or-flight response.

The physiological effects of anger don't end with the fight-or-flight response. Like the smoking habit, the anger habit can be hazardous to your health.

Dr. Redford Williams, a medical researcher at Duke University and coauthor (with his wife Virginia) of *Anger Kills*, reports that people who are "chronically angry" over everyday situations (traffic hassles, family hassles, job hassles) run a higher risk for heart disease and other illnesses. Chronic anger, he concludes, "raises your vulnerability to whatever pathogens you might be exposed to: a germ, a cold virus, or a familial predisposition to cancer or heart disease."[1]

Dr. Williams cites two studies that tracked the lives of medical and law students over a quarter of a century. Those studies revealed that twenty-five-year-old men who have a problem with chronic anger (as measured by psychological testing) are four to six times more likely to die by age fifty than those who don't. Another study by Harvard Medical School found that chronically angry men were three times as likely to develop coronary heart disease as those with low anger levels.[2] Anger is also linked to depression. Psychiatrists and psychologists often refer to depression as "anger turned inward."

To make matters worse, we frequently respond to anger with coping techniques that injure our health—drinking, drugging, overeating, or smoking. Ironically, this defense mechanism that was built into our makeup to protect us from harm often undermines our health and well-being.

Good and angry

Not all anger is harmful or destructive. There *is* such a thing as righteous indignation. There are times when anger is good and constructive. If it hadn't been for the anger of people like Martin Luther King, Jr., and Rosa Parks, African-Americans might still be living in a segregated society today. The civil rights movement of the 1960s was a movement of nonviolent anger, following the example of Mohandas Gandhi, who once said, "As heat conserved is transmuted into energy, even so our anger controlled can be transmuted into a power which can move the world."

During the Great Depression, writer John Steinbeck first became acquainted with the plight of California's migrant farm workers while researching a series of newspaper articles. He went to the camps and the fields. He watched the people work, listened to their stories, and felt their misery seeping into his own skin. He saw these people as noble, deserving human beings, exploited and crushed by a cruel and unfair world. What he saw angered him—and out of that anger came a great novel.

Steinbeck began writing *The Grapes of Wrath* in June 1938. It was not the first novel he had written, but he wanted it to be his greatest—and he wanted to write it quickly, so that the entire world would soon know of the injustices these workers suffered. Whenever he felt blocked or discouraged, he remembered the social evils he had witnessed—and his anger would surge and revitalize him. By October 1938, the book was finished—written in just five months, fueled by Steinbeck's righteous anger against injustice. *The Grapes of Wrath* became Steinbeck's masterpiece, winning him the Pulitzer Prize in 1940. It also became a force for change that helped improve conditions for California's migrant laborers and their families.

As Aristotle once observed, "We praise a man who feels angry on the right grounds and against the right persons and also in the right manner at the right moment and for the right length of time." Righteous indignation is not a brawling, raging fury. Anger against injustice must be controlled and focused. The purpose of this kind of anger is not to destroy people or property, but to restore justice. It is not a nasty, ill-tempered anger, but a compassionate, well-tempered anger. Handled in a healthy way, focused in the right direction, anger can be a beneficial part of our emotional makeup.

Taming the anger beast

The ability to manage our anger and control our behavior is critical to maintaining healthy relationships, both at home and in the workplace. Here are some suggestions for managing anger in a healthy way:

1. Adopt a forgiving attitude.

There was a time when I got as upset as anyone about obnoxious drivers. But I guess I'm making a little progress. Recently, I was in the middle lane of the freeway, driving at normal freeway speeds, taking my son to his percussion lesson. Suddenly, a black Dodge Viper swung around me on the left, pulled into my lane no more than ten feet in front of me, and hit the brakes. I had to brake so suddenly that my son and I were thrown against our seat restraints.

For a moment, I was livid. The guy could have caused a serious accident! I considered hitting my horn—then decided to let go of my anger. A few seconds later, I saw the guy's plan. He was making for an off-ramp just ahead, crossing from the far left lane to the far right lane. As soon as it was clear on the right, he made his move and lunged for the off-ramp.

Curious as to what sort of idiot would drive so recklessly, I glanced over at the driver as he was going up the off-ramp. He was a young male, about twenty. He looked back at me, smirking obnoxiously and *waving*. Being reckless wasn't enough for this guy. He had to be snotty to top it off.

Well, I had followed this guy for about a quarter of a mile, and that had given me time to settle my anger and think about how I wanted to respond. I had already made up my mind that I wanted to be a good example to my son. *Besides*, I thought to

> "*A*n emotion isn't good or bad, an emotion just is. Being angry may make us feel bad, it may be extremely unpleasant, but it is not "bad" or "wrong" to feel angry.

myself, *a guy who drives a Viper probably has some inadequacy issues regarding his testosterone levels.* So what did I do? I smiled and waved back (and yes, I waved with *all five* fingers).

He saw my wave and friendly smile—and the look on his face was priceless. His smile suddenly disappeared. He was so distracted, he nearly scraped the guardrail! The moral to the story: Don't let them get inside your head and mess with your emotions. Don't let them spoil your day. Forgive and move on.

2. Use your head (or, more precisely, your cerebral cortex).

As soon as you feel a surge of anger, *think*. Ask yourself: "Is my anger appropriate to the provocation—or am I overreacting? Will my anger make this situation better—or worse?" Anger is an unreasoning reaction that arises from the primitive parts of the brain. To control your anger, engage your reasoning ability and examine the situation calmly and rationally.

After an episode of uncontrolled rage, some people feel as if they were "beside themselves." A typical remorseful observation: "It was as if I were standing outside myself, watching this crazy person fly into a tirade—and that crazy person was me!" Perhaps there is a sense in which our cerebral cortex (the rational, thinking part of the brain) actually stands back and gazes with horror at what the more primitive parts of our brain drive us to do.

Although neuroscientists tell us there is no single "emotion center" in the brain, research shows that our emotional states primarily involve the areas of the *limbic system*. The primitive impulses of the limbic system are normally held in check by the thinking, reasoning cerebral cortex. But if the limbic system goes into overdrive, putting out waves of anger, stimulating the "fight-or-flight" response, the cerebral cortex can become overwhelmed, so that it no longer controls the animalistic urges of the primitive parts of the brain. Anger takes over and turns to aggression. And the rational brain can only watch helplessly as anger hijacks the personality like a terrorist hijacking an airplane.

It turns out there is good scientific and medical wisdom in Thomas Jefferson's adage: "When angry, count ten before you speak; if very angry, a hundred." Penelope Russianoff, psychologist and author of *When Am I Going to Be Happy?*, describes the physiological benefits of counting to ten when you first feel angry. She says that the external stimulus that produces feelings of anger reach the thalamus first (one of the primary emotional centers of the brain). There, the emotion of anger is triggered. "If we act on anger at that instant," observes Russianoff, "our response will be emotional, even violent. However, if we delay for just a few seconds, the thalamus can relay the message up to the cerebrum, the seat of logic and reason."[3]

The key to remaining in control, then, is to *use your head*. Pause, take a deep breath, count to ten, and think carefully about what is happening. Give the rational part of yourself time to regain control.

3. Take a reality check.

Talk through your anger with a trusted friend (ask, "Mind if I vent for a few minutes?"). Make sure your friend can be trusted to keep a confidence. It also helps if this person has the wisdom and maturity to help you sort out your feelings. You want to vent with a friend who can help you "reality check" your emotions, sorting out the reasonable from the irrational.

4. Get physical.

Doing something active is a safe, nonaggressive way to work off angry emotions. Take a walk or a jog. Work in the garden or clean house. You can even commit some harmless mayhem, like punching a pillow. Avoid punching walls or doors or doing anything that could hurt yourself or others. Because anger triggers "fight-or-flight" chemicals in your body, you have a lot of aggressive energy bottled up inside you.

Let it out safely, and when you are done, you will probably have greater control over your emotions.

5. Write down your anger.

Express your feelings in a diary or journal. Or better yet, just write them on a piece of paper, then burn the paper. (Do you really need to keep those thoughts around after you've expressed them? Probably not.) Sometimes just setting your feelings down on paper is sufficient to get all the emotional poisons out of your system.

6. Make a careful, conscious choice as to how you will respond to feelings of anger.

Some years ago, while working with a group of psychiatrists and psychologists on a 600-page self-help book called *The Complete Life Encyclopedia*, I learned that people generally choose one of four responses to the emotion of anger:

> Suppression
> Open aggression
> Passive aggression
> Assertive expression

The first three approaches are unhealthy approaches. The fourth— assertive expression of anger—is the only healthy approach. Let's look at them:

First, **suppression**. People who suppress their anger were usually trained from childhood to see emotions as unacceptable. As a result, they do not accept their feelings as valid. They conclude, "My feelings don't matter enough to be expressed." Thinking that anger is "bad," they retreat into denial: "Me? Angry? What makes you think I'm angry?"

Some suppress their anger in a smug and superior way: "I'm not angry, I'm in control. *You* are the one with the anger problem, not me." Such people often hold rigid beliefs, including inflexible religious beliefs. Being "right" is very important to them, and they suppress their anger because they see anger as a flaw; blowing up would cause them to lose face.

Suppressing doesn't eliminate anger—it only drives hostile emotions underground, where they fester into bitterness. A lifetime of suppressed anger tends to produce a twisted, ugly personality.

Second, **open aggression**. This is what most people think of when they hear the word *anger*: rage, shouting, intimidation, even violence. Open aggression is a self-centered response to feelings of anger. The person who explodes in anger cares only for his own wants and feelings; he sends a message loud and clear: "You and your feelings don't matter to me. I don't care who I hurt."

The openly aggressive person is often insecure. By being loud, pounding the table, and making bigger, more violent gestures and facial expressions, the insecure person makes himself louder and "larger" in order to be heard and obeyed. People who operate consistently from open aggression eventually destroy their most important relationships—and their own reputations.

Some people have the mistaken idea that "expressing" their anger through open aggression is healthy, that it gets the anger out of you. In reality, the "expression" of anger through open aggression actually seems to stimulate the primitive emotional regions of the brain, causing anger to breed *more* anger. That is why open aggression easily spirals out of control, escalating rapidly from verbal abuse to physical violence. Once the primitive emotional centers of the brain wrest control away from the rational part of the brain, it is easy for anger to transmute into a violent rage.

Third, **passive aggression**. This response to anger is destructive, like open aggression, but it operates secretly and indirectly instead of openly. Examples of passive aggressive behavior:

- Muttering under your breath ("*Mutter-mutter!*" "What did you say?!" "Who, innocent little me? I didn't say a thing!")

- Showing up late or stalling when the other person is rushed.

- Someone asks you to do something, you grudgingly say, "Okay," then you "forget" to do it ("Heh-heh-heh!").

- Joking in a hurtful way, then when the other person gets offended, you say, "Gee, can't you take a joke?"

- Being friendly to a person's face then sabotaging her behind her back.

The passive aggressive approach is a way to control people and situations without appearing to be in control. It is adopted by people who don't feel competent to express their anger openly. Passive aggressors have an uncanny knack for pushing other people's buttons. They get others riled while remaining outwardly calm, making other people look like the aggressors. Like those who suppress anger, passive aggressors usually deny being angry—but the anger is there, all right.

Psychologist Jim Osterhaus uses naval warfare as a metaphor to describe the difference between open aggression and passive aggression. "Open aggression," he once told me, "is like a battleship that turns broadside to the target and unleashes a barrage from its sixteen-inch guns. Passive aggression is like a submarine that rises to periscope depth, fires a spread of torpedoes, then disappears before the torpedoes hit their target. Passive aggression can be as destructive as open aggression, but it is much more sneaky. It is sabotage instead of frontal assault."

> "Some people have the mistaken idea that 'expressing' their anger through open aggression is healthy, that it gets the anger out of you."

Fourth, *assertive expression*. All of the preceding responses are unhealthy and destructive. But now we come to the one *healthy* response to anger. The assertive but nonaggressive expression of anger is a sign of emotional maturity. When we talk out our anger in an assertive but nonaggressive way, we show that our feelings matter—but we also respect the feelings of the other person: "I'm angry about this situation, but I also care about you and about your feelings. Let's solve this problem together."

To be assertive doesn't mean to be pushy or abrasive; it simply means that we state our thoughts and emotions firmly and fairly, and with consideration for the other person. Assertiveness has to do with the way you verbalize your anger. It is possible to say, "I felt angry when you did such and such," without raising your voice, pounding a wall, or any of the other actions that usually accompany aggressive anger. Assertiveness is anger under control. It is reasoned, rational anger. It is honest but caring.

If, while discussing your anger, you sense the other person becoming heated, you can defuse the situation by listening calmly and responding with a lowered voice. This goes against the animalistic urges that arise from the primitive limbic system—the animal part of you will naturally want to respond with aggression and intimidation. But just remember: You are a human being, with a reasoning cerebral cortex. Use your rational mind to stay out of the aggressive mode and in the controlled, assertive mode.

"Rivers of rage..."

Christopher Scanlon, the writer of "Daddy's Rage," went on to describe how he came to understand and better control his anger. After one of his tirades left his three daughters crying, his wife issued an ultimatum: The rage had to stop—or Scanlon would lose his family.

So Christopher Scanlon decided to approach this problem the way he approached most of the important issues in his life: He would write about it. He began keeping a "Temper Log," in which he journaled his emotional struggles, job stresses, financial worries, and family worries. As he journaled, patterns began to emerge: He discovered that there were certain times when he was most likely to lose his temper—in the morning, during the rush to get off to work, and in the evenings, after a tiring day and a ride home on the Metro. By becoming more conscious of those vulnerable times, he learned to take control of his anger.

Scanlon also realized that he had been responding to anger with the style that was modeled for him in childhood. His father was an embittered alcoholic who often came home drunk. One of Scanlon's few early memories is of a horrible argument between his father and mother. His dad had been out of work for weeks, he had been drinking, and he came home to find his wife at the kitchen table, praying for him. He flew into a rage. "If your God is so good," he roared, "why are the sheriffs coming to the door about the bills I can't pay? Why am I broke? Why can't I find a job?....Why, dammit? Why?" Then he grasped his wife's rosary and tore it from her hands. Scanlon recalls hearing the beads of the rosary "dancing like marbles on the linoleum."

While all this was going on, young Christopher Scanlon and his brother were crying in their bedroom. Suddenly, the door of their room was flung open. Scanlon recalls, "In the placid cruelty of what passes for reason in a drunk's mind, he told us, 'Don't worry boys, your mother and I are getting a divorce,' which, of course, sent our wails even higher."

Not that Christopher Scanlon blames his own anger on his father. He takes full responsibility for his own behavior. Accepting responsibility, of course, is the first step in changing one's behavior. The memory of his father's anger helps to keep Scanlon's own anger in check. He concludes:

> I meet my father now in the dark of my children's bedroom, hearing in my shouts the echoes of his rage, the legacy of anger passed from father to son.... Rivers of rage run from one generation to another, and it may be impossible to staunch the flow. But I have to keep trying. One breakfast, one bedtime, one day at a time.[4]

Next to love, anger is the most powerful of all human emotions. Uncontrolled, it becomes a force of unimaginable destruction, capable of taking away from us everything we value—family, career, reputation. But controlled, channeled, and surrounded by love, anger can become a tool for growth and understanding. The choice is yours.

Do I Have to Forgive Others?

Just a few days before Christmas 1974, ten-year-old Chris Carrier stepped off the school bus a few blocks from his home in Coral Gables, Florida. A man was waiting for the boy at the bus stop. He called Chris by name and the boy saw no reason not to accept a ride home with the man.

That was the last anyone saw of Chris Carrier for six days.

During those six days, the boy's disappearance made national headlines. The day after Christmas, a hunter found the boy sitting on a rock in the Everglades, about seventy-five miles from home. He was dazed, bruised, and bleeding. The kidnapper had tortured the boy, burning his skin with cigarettes, and had stabbed him in the chest with an ice pick. Then he had put a gun to Chris's head and shot him in the right temple. The bullet went through his head, exiting the left temple. Amazingly, Chris survived, though he lost the sight in his left eye.

The police quickly zeroed in on David McAllister, a male nurse in his mid-fifties who had taken care of an elderly member of the Carrier family. Significantly, Chris's father, Hugh Carrier, had terminated McAllister for drinking on the job six months before.

McAllister had a criminal record and closely resembled a composite sketch drawn from eyewitness descriptions. But the police had no physical evidence to conclusively link McAllister to the crime. He was never charged.

Chris Carrier suffered from the trauma of his ordeal. "Ages ten to thirteen were three years of insecurity," he later recalled. "At night, if I heard the floorboards creak, I'd get up and sleep at the foot of my parents' bed. I was constantly afraid of what was around the next corner." At thirteen, Chris Carrier had a spiritual epiphany. "From that point," he recalled, "I started saying, 'It's time to get on with my life.'" He grew up and married, and he and his wife, Leslie, had two children. Whenever anyone heard his story, the question arose, "What would you do if you met the man who kidnapped you?" It was a question he couldn't answer.

In September 1996, his phone rang. It was Charles Scherer, the police detective who had worked the case. The unresolved kidnapping had bothered Scherer for years; he was convinced McAllister was guilty. Finally, years after the statute of limitations had run out, Scherer learned that McAllister was at Greynolds Park Manor, a North Miami Beach nursing home. At seventy-seven, McAllister was frail, blind, and dying. Scherer asked Chris if he would meet with McAllister. Chris agreed.

On Labor Day weekend 1996, Chris Carrier and his pastor sat down at McAllister's bedside. It was a difficult meeting. McAllister was reluctant to admit anything. Finally, he did admit to the kidnapping, but not the shooting. Carrier's pastor asked, "Would you like to say you're sorry to the boy?"

"I wish I could," said the old man.

"Here he is," said the pastor. "He's listening."

In a few halting words, McAllister apologized—and he began to cry. Chris told the old man he forgave him.

Over the next few weeks, Chris Carrier continued to go to the convalescent home and visit with McAllister. He read to him and talked with him. He took his wife and daughters to meet him, to show McAllister that his life had turned out well. The two men—once kidnapper and victim—became friends.

The great irony is that while the victim had gotten on with his life, the perpetrator had remained in a self-made emotional prison for twenty-two years. "He's never been able to live without memories and pain," Carrier observed. "He has paid his price, served his time."

On September 26, 1996, Chris Carrier went to the nursing home for a visit—their last, as it turned out. He took along some smoked amberjack fish and shared it with McAllister. They talked for a while, and before he left, Chris made sure that McAllister was warm and comfortable. A few hours later, McAllister died.[1]

Ask yourself, if you had gone through what Chris Carrier did, would you be able to forgive David McAllister? Fortunately, few of us will ever be placed in such an extreme situation, but one thing is sure: The way

Chris Carrier chose to respond is the healthiest and most positive way to live. A person who is able to *forgive* is able to truly *live*.

Forgiveness is good medicine

Everett Worthington, a Virginia psychologist and director of the Templeton Foundation for Forgiveness Research, says people who hold back forgiveness tend to marinate in anger and hostility—deadly emotional poisons that contribute to arteriosclerosis, heart attacks, and strokes. An unforgiving personality is subject to greater stress, which weakens the immune system, making a person more susceptible to various diseases, including cancer. People who cannot or will not forgive are also more prone to such emotional problems as anxiety and depression.[2]

The issue of forgiveness is not a theoretical issue for Dr. Worthington. In 1996, shortly after he finished writing *To Forgive Is Human: How to Put Your Past in the Past* (with coauthors Michael E. McCullough and Steven Sandage), he learned that his seventy-eight-year-old mother, Frances, had been beaten to death by an intruder in her Knoxville, Tennessee, home. No arrest was ever made. Thinking back to the brutal tragedy, Dr. Worthington says, "I looked at a baseball bat and said, 'I wish I could have that guy here. I'd beat his brains out.' Then I thought, 'Whose heart is darker?'" Today, he says he has no hate for the anonymous killer.[3]

Most people regard forgiveness as a moral or spiritual issue, a matter of the soul. And, of course, it is. But science has shown that forgiveness is not only the *right* thing to do—it is also the *healthy* thing to do. The act of forgiveness benefits the body as well as the soul. Forgiveness is good medicine, making you a healthier and happier person.

What forgiveness is—and is not

Let's define what we mean by forgiveness: *Forgiveness is a choice to renounce anger or resentment against an offender.* It is a decision we make—not an emotion we feel. Feelings come and go, but if we make a *decision*, we can *will* ourselves to abide by that decision, despite our wavering feelings.

There is an old cliché, "Forgive and forget." But you and I both know that when someone has hurt us deeply, it is impossible to forget. We can't simply press a "delete" button on our memories. In fact, our brains are constructed in such a way that the most painful memories tend to be the ones that are the most permanently imprinted. So forgetting is *not* a component of forgiving. Fact is, we must forgive precisely because it is *impossible* to forget. The memory of the hurt will come back to us again and again, so we must make a deliberate choice to renounce anger and resentment. If we don't, we will stay mired in bitterness, rage, and hatred.

Many people see forgiveness as a sign of weakness. They may *feel* stronger and more powerful when they hold onto a grudge, but in reality holding grudges is nothing more than doing what comes naturally. Hating is easy. Forgiving is hard. The act of forgiveness takes enormous strength of will, and even great courage. Only those who are mentally, emotionally, and spiritually *tough* are able to forgive, because forgiveness saws across the grain of your emotions. *Forgiveness is not for wimps.*

Remember our definition of forgiveness: a choice to renounce anger or resentment against an offender. From this definition, we get a sense of what forgiveness is—and what it is not. Forgiveness doesn't mean that we tolerate bad behavior. It doesn't mean that we condone or excuse evil acts. It doesn't mean there are no consequences for the offender. It doesn't mean a lawbreaker shouldn't be brought to justice. It doesn't even mean that we have to reconcile, be friends with, or like the offender. It simply means that we give up our anger and resentment. Those feelings will come back to us again and again, but instead of wallowing in them, we say, "I choose not to be angry and bitter. I'm going to mentally change the subject. I've made a decision to forgive, and I'm sticking to it."

If a friend seriously or repeatedly betrays you, it is possible to forgive without remaining friends with that person. You can say, "I forgive you, I have let go of my anger toward you—but at the same time, I can see that it's not good for me to have you in my life. So I can no longer be your friend."

Unfortunately, a lot of people can't tell the difference between forgiveness and excusing evil. After two teenage gunmen killed twelve students and a teacher, plus themselves, at Columbine High School near Denver, a local carpenter erected a memorial to the dead on a bluff overlooking the school. The memorial consisted of fifteen wooden crosses, thirteen for the victims, two for the perpetrators. At the base of the cross of one of the killers, someone had placed the message, "Forgive them, Lord, they know not what they do."

Should we forgive them? Should the parents, brothers, and sisters of the slain students forgive them? Should the widow and children of the slain teacher forgive them? The father and stepfather of one of the murdered students didn't think so. They went to the bluff, pulled the two crosses out of the ground, and chopped them into kindling.

It would be so easy to say, "Forgive them"—as long as it wasn't *your* son or *your* daughter or *your* husband or *your* father who was murdered. But when you have just put a loved one in the ground, talk of "forgiving" the killers sounds like an obscenity, like a betrayal of the dead. It is as if we are saying that a murder victim's life has so little value that we can say to the murderer, "You're excused."

> "*F*orgiveness is not for wimps."

There is a kind of forgiveness that I call *evil forgiveness*. Does that term sound too strong? How can forgiveness ever be "evil"? I assure you, I chose those words with care and precision. I believe it is a terrible, destructive act to offer a glib, shallow kind of "forgiveness" that simply excuses evil as if it did not exist. Despite what may seem to be good intentions, we cause enormous harm to innocent people when we excuse evil and give license to the guilty.

I have had conversations (perhaps you have, too) with people who say, "I'm a forgiving person, and I believe we should forgive this mass murderer or this serial child molester. He doesn't need our condemnation—he needs our understanding. Why can't everyone be as forgiving as I am?" By "forgiving" a wrong that was never done to them, these people set themselves up as morally superior to those who cannot or will not "forgive" as readily as they do. The scary thing is that such people have a tendency to end up on juries, where they "forgive" dangerous repeat criminals and turn them loose on society. That kind of false "forgiveness," no matter how well-intentioned, has a destructive effect on all of us. That is why I call it *evil forgiveness*.

If someone burns down your house, what right do I have to go to the arsonist and say, "I forgive you"? It wasn't my house he burned down; it was yours. You and only you have the right to forgive that person. If some uninvolved bystander "forgives" an evil that was done to you, that bystander is setting himself up as God and judge. If you aren't personally injured by another person's actions, then you are not in a position to forgive.

Simon Wiesenthal was a young architect working in Lvov, Poland, when the country was invaded by the Nazis in 1939. From 1941 to 1945, he was interned in several concentration camps, including Buchenwald and Mauthausen. In his 1969 book *The Sunflower: On the Possibilities and Limits of Forgiveness*, he describes an incident at Mauthausen. One day, he was called out of a labor detail and taken to a hospital. There a wounded Nazi soldier named Karl lay dying. As his last request, the soldier had asked that a Jew be brought to him from the camp to hear his confession and give him absolution. So Wiesenthal was the Jew they chose. Wiesenthal listened as the soldier confessed to a number of horrible atrocities, including the butchering of a Jewish family with a small child. When the soldier had finished speaking, Wiesenthal turned and left the room without a word.

Simon Wiesenthal gave the soldier no forgiveness, no absolution. It wasn't his to give. It may seem harsh, but the moral to this story is clear: It is arrogant and morally offensive to forgive what is not ours to forgive. True forgiveness does not condone evil. It looks evil square in the eye, calls it what it is, and holds people accountable for their actions—not in an angry or resentful way, but honestly and objectively. In fact, holding people accountable should be a loving and forgiving act. It is something you do for a person's own good, in order to motivate positive change.

The primary purpose of forgiveness is not to set offenders free from the consequences of their actions. It is to set us free from anger and bitterness, so we can get on with our lives.

How to forgive

Dr. Worthington believes that anyone who wants to forgive can forgive. Having chosen to let go of anger and bitterness toward the intruder who murdered his own mother, he speaks with authority. He offers a five-step approach to forgiveness called REACH—an acronym for:

R — Recall the hurt. Objectively accept the fact that an offense was done to you—but do so without blaming or bitterness.

E — Empathize with the offender. Try to see the situation from his or her point of view. Forgiveness becomes easier if we can step into the offender's shoes, even for a moment. Dr. Worthington explains how he himself took this step: "I tried to imagine the guy who broke into my mother's house. He doesn't expect anyone to be home; when he hears someone behind him, he just reacts."

A — Altruism—that is, give an altruistic gift of forgiveness. Dr. Worthington suggests that you think of a time you hurt someone else and were forgiven; try to recall how it felt. Then give that same gift to someone in your own life.

C — Commit yourself to the decision you have made. Confide this decision to a friend or write a letter of forgiveness to the offender (but don't mail it). This, says Dr. Worthington, will help to seal your decision.

H — Hold on to your decision to forgive. The memory of the offense will come back to you, along with feelings of anger and resentment. That's normal. It doesn't mean you haven't forgiven. It just means you're human. When that happens, renew your decision to forgive. Each time you do so, it will become easier. Eventually, resentment will lose its power over you.

If you are religiously inclined, you may want to add another step to Dr. Worthington's REACH formula: Prayer. (If you make this Step 1, then the acronym REACH becomes PREACH.) Many people with a strong belief in a Higher Power find that prayer and meditation lends added strength to their effort to forgive.

Forgiveness versus reconciliation

In most cases, forgiveness will lead to reconciliation between you and the offender. In extreme cases, you may have to forgive without restoring the relationship. For example, if your marriage partner cheats on you—especially if unfaithfulness is a pattern—it may not be healthy or smart for you to take this person back into your life. But even if you don't reconcile, forgive. Let go of the bitterness of betrayal—not to do your straying partner any favors, but to do yourself a favor. You don't want to stay locked in an emotional death-struggle with this person. You want to be free. And the only way to be free is to forgive.

However, if, in an extreme case, you do choose to reconcile with the offender, I recommend certain basic conditions. Someone has called these conditions "The Four Rs of Reconciliation." They are:

1. The offender must accept *responsibility* for what he or she did. There can be no reconciliation until the offender admits that the act was wrong and accepts responsibility without excuses or evasions.

2. The offender must demonstrate authentic *remorse* for what he or

she did. You can be sure a person is not genuinely remorseful when he snarls, "Awright, awright, if it makes you feel better, I'm sorry! Geez, get off my back!" A remorseful person is not defensive or angry at being caught. He is profoundly heartbroken over having hurt you.

3. The offender must demonstrate true *repentance*. To repent means to turn around and move in a new direction.

4. The offender must *repair* the damage he has caused—at least, as much as possible. The person who damaged your reputation should go to every person he's told and set the record straight. The adulterer should be willing to completely cut all ties with the illicit lover and accept restrictions on his time and whereabouts so that trust can be rebuilt. The person who stole from you should be willing to make full restitution if it takes a lifetime.

These are the basic requirements for reconciliation. Understand, reconciliation isn't easy; in fact, it's not always possible. But even if you are never able to reconcile with the person who hurt you, you can still forgive. You have a life to live, and only a finite number of moments in which to live it. Don't waste a single moment dwelling on bitterness.

Forgiveness is not something you do for anyone else. It's something you do for you.

10

How Can I Forgive Myself?

"Most of my life has been ruled by guilt," actress Grace Lee Whitney once told me.

When Grace was seven, her mother took her aside and told her she was an adopted child. Unfortunately, Grace didn't focus on the fact that she had been *chosen* by her adoptive parents. Instead, she focused on the fact that she had been (as she thought) "rejected" by her birth mother. Adoption is a wonderful gift to give a child, but Grace mistakenly assumed that her birth mother gave her up because there was something "wrong" with her.

Grace acted out her pain and self-hate by drinking and becoming sexually active by age thirteen. At age fourteen, she took her parents' car for a drunken joyride. As she drove along Grand River Avenue in Detroit, a man stepped into the street in front of her. Grace had no time to react, and the man went down beneath her wheels. She didn't even look back—and she was never caught. As far as she knows, she killed the man.

Growing up, she caused her parents enormous grief. As soon as she could strike out on her own, she left home to start a singing career. She married a drummer while a radio singer with the Ray Noble Orchestra; soon afterwards, she appeared on the *You Bet Your Life* comedy quiz show with Groucho Marx. She talked about her wedding while chatting with Groucho. Her parents happened to be watching the show that night— and that's how they learned of her marriage.

Grace went on to acting roles in various films and TV shows, eventually landing the role of Yeoman Rand on the original *Star Trek* series. "I felt a lot of guilt when I began filming *Star Trek*," she told me.

"Guilt about what?" I asked.

"I had begun sabotaging my marriage," she said. "I thought my marriage was holding back my career, so I tossed out my husband and filed for divorce. I felt guilty about destroying my nest and hurting my two boys. So I did a lot of drinking to deaden the immorality and self-hate. Then, when I was drinking, I did immoral things and I hated myself for it. So I felt more guilt, followed by more drinking to deaden the guilt.

"That's the way alcoholics live. You wake up and remember what you did the night before, and the guilt sets in. Or you wake up in a motel room and think, *What am I doing here? I don't even remember how I got here!* And you just feel awful. You feel like a terrible, bad person. Then you reach for another drink to make those feelings go away."

After being sexually assaulted by a Desilu producer and tossed off the show midway through the first season, Grace went into a deadly spiral of self-destructive drinking. There were times she would stop drinking for months—she calls it being a "dry drunk." She would replace booze with marijuana or some other substance, but her alcoholism was still progressing all the same. It was during one of Grace's "dry drunk" spells that her father was admitted to Veterans Hospital in Los Angeles.

"I had always thought of my dad as a rigid perfectionist," Grace recalled. "He would never let me forget that one B in a report card full of A's—and I resented it. Over the years, I had hurt him and my mother deeply, yet my dad would have done anything for me. It wasn't until he was in the hospital, dying of bacterial endocarditis, that I finally realized how much he loved me, and how much I loved him."

During the last few weeks of her father's life, Grace spent a lot of time at the hospital, talking to her dad, getting closer than they had ever been before. But then, as the end approached, he was placed on a respirator. "He could no longer talk," she explained. "They had a tube down his throat, and he fought it. It was horrible, and I couldn't stand to be there anymore, watching him struggle for life on death row. So I stopped going to see him."

The day her father died, Grace sat in the hospital lobby while her mother and her son, Scott, went to be with him. "I couldn't go up to his room," she told me. "I was in such pain, I just couldn't function. After a while, my mother came down and said, 'Grace, you have to go up there and say good-bye to your father—they're going to take him off the respirator.' I said, 'I can't!' Then my mother said something that would haunt me for a long time: 'Grace, if you don't go up there and say good-bye to your father, you're going to regret it for the rest of your life.'

"I felt horribly guilty—but I still couldn't go. My mother went back to his room without me. She and Scott were with my father when they took out the respirator tube. When he died, I was outside the hospital, sitting behind the bushes by the front steps, smoking a joint. The guilt I carried for years afterwards was almost more than I could bear."

It would be years before Grace would discover the solution to her guilt.

Appropriate and inappropriate guilt

My friend Dru Scott once defined guilt as "a feeling of deviation from a relevant standard."[1] We all have standards we try to live up to. And, being human, we all deviate from those standards from time to time. When the standard we set for ourselves is appropriate, realistic, and relevant to our lives, the guilt we feel when we deviate from that standard is accurate and realistic. We *should* feel guilty when we veer away from an appropriate standard. But if we set a standard that is unrealistically high, then the guilt we feel may be *inappropriate* or *false* guilt.

It's inappropriate to feel guilty about having a slightly messy house when you've got a preschooler to care for all day. It's inappropriate to feel guilty about not having the body of a supermodel or an Olympic athlete. Some people feel guilty if they are not being frantically busy every moment of the day. Others feel guilty about enjoying life while a friend is going through a tough time. These are all examples of inappropriate guilt.

Obsessive perfectionism is a common source of inappropriate guilt. Perfectionists tend to be guilt-driven workaholics who never feel they have done enough. They are often critical of themselves, judgmental toward others, and plagued by worry and guilt. They set themselves up for failure by imposing standards and expectations on themselves that are impossible to meet. Perfection cannot be achieved by any human being—but the perfectionist will keep trying, keep failing, and keep feeling guilty.

Are there people who never feel guilty? Of course there are. They're called *sociopaths*—people without a conscience. Many criminals have sociopathic personalities. They can lie, cheat, steal, and kill without a second thought, and they will never lose a moment's sleep over it. In fact, many sociopaths not only feel no guilt, they actually feel *good* about doing evil.

Ironically, only decent people are capable of feeling guilt. In fact, decent people frequently feel guilty for doing the *right* thing! They feel terrible when disciplining their children, because they love their children and want them to be happy. Decent people usually feel terribly conflicted when sitting on a jury, having to impose a verdict on a lawbreaker. Decent people feel guilty about asking for money that's owed them or asking people to stop talking in the theater while the movie is playing. Much of the guilt that decent people feel is *false* guilt.

> "*I*ronically, only decent people are capable of feeling guilt. In fact, decent people frequently feel guilty for doing the right thing!"

There is, of course, such a thing as *authentic* guilt. When we do something hurtful to ourselves or others, authentic guilt nags at us, telling us we've gotten offtrack. The purpose of authentic guilt is to get our attention so we can get back on course. Unfortunately, false guilt often shouts at us so loudly that we can't hear the voice of healthy guilt.

Hypothetical example: As a boy, David was continually told by his father that he was lazy and he'd never amount to anything. As a result, David is now a driven workaholic. He makes a ton of money and has become a hugely successful businessman—but his overachievement is driven by the guilt messages from childhood. He lives his entire life in an unconscious effort to prove his father wrong, to prove that he's *not* lazy and that he *will* amount to something. David's father died years ago, so David can never win his father's approval—yet he vainly keeps trying.

At the same time, David's marriage is on the verge of collapse. He's never home, he's always at the office, and his two children scarcely recognize him. When his wife confronts him about the fact that he is neglecting his family, he denies it. "Neglecting my family!" he objects. "Look at this home! We've got a Lexus and a Mercedes in the driveway, a membership at the club, private schools for the kids—what more could a family want?"

"How about a father who comes home at night?" asks his wife.

But David won't hear it. He *can't* hear it. His false guilt, inflicted on him by a now-dead father, drowns out the real guilt he should feel for neglecting his family.

Five steps to eliminating guilt

The obvious question is: How do we tell the difference between authentic guilt and false guilt?

Consider Dru Scott's definition of guilt: "a feeling of deviation from a relevant standard." Now ask yourself: "What do I feel guilty about?" Clearly define in your mind what it is that drives guilt feelings. Then ask yourself: "What relevant standard have I violated?" Maybe you have deviated from a moral standard set for you by your religious beliefs. Or maybe you have deviated from a standard set for you by your parents, by society, or by peer pressure. Get it very clear in your mind what you have done (or failed to do) and what standard this act or omission violates. It may be helpful to write it down on a piece of paper or discuss your guilt feelings with a friend. This helps get your feelings out where they can be objectively analyzed.

Now ask yourself: "Did the thing I did (or failed to do) violate a *relevant* standard for my life? Did I truly deviate from my own moral values, my own sense of right and wrong? Or did I merely violate some irrelevant and unimportant standard, a standard that other people—my parents, my society, my peers—set for me?" If you did not violate a *relevant* standard for your life, your feelings are probably *false* guilt. The simple act of recognizing false guilt may enable you move beyond those feelings.

But what if it is *authentic* guilt you feel? Then you must resolve your guilt in a healthy way. Here are some steps for resolving that guilt.

1. Make a habit of regular moral self-examination.

We should examine our souls on a daily basis. If you are religiously inclined, this can take place during a daily prayer and meditation time in the morning or evening. Before going to sleep at night, you might like to mentally replay the day, recalling your actions toward others, pondering what you could have done better or if there are people you might have wronged.

Seven of the Twelve Steps of Alcoholics Anonymous have to do with moral self-examination. Some examples: Step 4, "Made a searching and fearless moral inventory of ourselves." Step 5, "Admitted to God, to ourselves, and to another human being the exact nature of our wrongs." Step 8. "Made a list of all persons we had harmed, and became willing to make amends to them all."

I have found it helpful to meet regularly with a small group of friends with whom I can be open and honest and who will be honest with me about what they see in my life. These groups can take various forms, such as support groups, recovery groups, or accountability groups. The important thing is to have a few close friends who care enough to help you penetrate your denial and defensiveness, so your faults can be admitted and corrected.

2. Apologize.

When you apologize to someone you've wronged, you accept the fact that you were wrong and open your soul to receive absolution, so that your guilt can be removed from the record. When you apologize, especially if you are not sure how your apology will be received, I recommend you say, "I'm sorry," not "Please forgive me." When you say, "I'm sorry" to someone, you give the gift of an apology to that person. True, it is only what you owe that person—but it is still a gift. If the other person chooses to stay angry and unforgiving, at least the apology has been given, and you have done what you needed to do.

But if you say, "Please forgive me," you are not giving a gift, you are making a request—and a request can be denied. What happens to you if that person spurns your request? You'll feel even worse than before. The purpose of an apology is not to put you in the position of a beggar, pleading for mercy. The purpose of an apology is to demonstrate your sorrow and remorse. So don't make a request; give a gift. And once the gift is given, leave it there. It is up to the other person to accept the gift or not—but at least you have accomplished what you set out to do.

This is not to say that the words "I'm sorry" are necessarily a complete apology. If you accidentally step on someone's foot, then "I'm sorry" pretty well covers it. But when you have committed a serious offense, such as breaching a trust, betraying a confidence, damaging a relationship, or committing a serious moral transgression, it is important that you make a serious, detailed apology in which you:

- Take full responsibility for what you did. Don't make excuses. Don't minimize what you did. Don't blame anyone else. Don't call it a "mistake." Say, "It was my fault, and it was wrong."

- Acknowledge that what you did was hurtful to the person you offended. Make it clear that you realize the consequences of your action and how this has made the other person feel.

- Express your commitment to change your behavior in the future.

Whatever you do, demonstrate total sincerity and humility. As G.K. Chesterton observed, "A stiff apology is a second insult....The injured party does not want to be compensated because he has been wronged; he wants to be healed because he has been hurt."

3. Make amends.

When you have offended another person, an apology may not be enough. You may need to make amends. That means doing whatever you can to make a wrong situation right—or as close to right as possible. Obviously, not all wrongs can be righted. But making amends is at least a step or two in the right direction. The word amend means to compensate (or offer compensation), to make reparation, or to make restitution. Making amends visibly demonstrates the reality of your remorse. Words are cheap, but amends are costly.

4. Lean on your spirituality.

Up to this point, we've been talking about practical rather than spiritual approaches to resolving guilt—but we should not neglect the spiritual dimension. Clearly, it is not the purpose of this book to point you to a particular religion or spiritual path. However, the spiritual component of your life *can* play a significant role in resolving guilt feelings. The world's great religions present God as the one who offers forgiveness and release from guilt. As actress Grace Lee Whitney once told me, "Alcohol could numb my guilt for a night—but only God could get rid of my guilt for good." For some people, guilt creates a sense of separation and estrangement from God. If guilt is the result of a spiritual *dis*connect, then it is only logical that the ultimate solution for guilt is to reestablish a spiritual connection.

5. Forgive yourself.

It is just as important to forgive yourself as it is to forgive others. Forgiving yourself does not mean pretending it never happened. Forgiveness (whether of yourself or someone else) always begins with a clear-eyed recognition of the wrong that was done. It begins with the awful fact that you have done something that makes you feel disappointed or even angry with yourself.

If you have a hard time forgiving yourself, ask yourself this question: "Could I forgive someone else for doing what I did? If a friend of mine did what I did, would I despise her—or forgive her?" Many people are much harder on themselves than on other people. Sometimes it helps to step outside of yourself, look at yourself objectively, and say, "What I did was wrong, but it was human—and it is forgivable. I'm making a decision to forgive and accept myself."

Guilt is like an alarm clock. It's supposed to wake us up and prod us to action. When your alarm clock sounds in the morning, what do you do? Well, the theory behind alarm clocks is that you shut off the alarm, get out of bed, and start the day. But suppose that, instead of shutting off the alarm and getting up, you just lie in bed, listening to the alarm. "Oh, that alarm sounds terrible," you say to yourself. "It makes me feel so bad. I wish that alarm would just be quiet, but it keeps going on and on!"

A lot of us respond to guilt that way. Instead of shutting off the alarm of guilt and making constructive changes in our lives, we just lie there and listen to it buzz. That alarm is ringing for a purpose. It is telling you to get up and get your life in order. How will you answer it? Maybe you need to spend more time with your family. Maybe you need to mend fences with a neighbor or coworker. Maybe you need to deal with an addiction problem. Maybe you need to stop lying or cheating in your business. Whatever it is, shut off the alarm, get up, and get your life on track.

Life after guilt

But what do you do with guilt feelings when there is no way to apologize, no way to make amends, because the person you hurt is no longer living? That's the situation Grace Lee Whitney faced after the death of her father. She let her father die without saying a final "I love you"—and the guilt she felt continued to eat her alive even after she got clean and sober.

After getting into recovery for alcoholism, Grace knew that one reason she drank was to anesthetize the pain of her guilt. So if she was going to keep her sobriety, she had to get rid of the guilt. She explained to me the process she went through to resolve years and years of accumulated guilt.

> "It is just as important to forgive yourself as it is to forgive others."

"Step 8 of the Twelve Steps," she told me, "says that we have 'made a list of all persons we had harmed, and became willing to make amends to them all.' I had a lot of people to make amends to. So I wrote a personal inventory—*seventy-eight pages* detailing all the pain I'd caused other people, all the places I turned left when I should have turned right.

"I knew I had to begin with my parents. I had hurt them both deeply. So, a year and a half into my sobriety, I made amends to my mother. I went down on my knees in front of her, and I didn't get up from my knees until I had listed every sin I had committed against her. Then I asked her forgiveness for all the pain I had caused her over the years—for being such a difficult child, for marrying without even telling her about it, for all my drunkenness and sexaholism. And she forgave me."

But what about Grace's father? How do you receive forgiveness from the dead?

"I was in a recovery meeting," Grace told me, "talking about how I had never said good-bye to my father. And it hit me how incredibly self-centered I had been—smoking a joint instead of saying good-bye to my father. And I just came unglued. I couldn't stop crying. I said, 'The worst of it is that there's nothing I can do to make it up to him!'"

But the other people in the group told her, "No, there *is* something you can do. You can write a love letter to your father, then take it to his grave and read it to him."

Well, that had never occurred to her—but it made sense. So she wrote out a letter to her father, a long inventory of all the ways she had hurt him from the time she was a child to the day of his death. Then she went to his grave and sat down in the grass next to his headstone. There, for the next hour and a half, she read the letter and poured out her heart to her father. Then she said, "Daddy, I'm so sorry. I know how much I hurt you. I know you loved me and you put up with a lot from me. And I want you to know I love you, too."

Finally, when all her tears and grief and guilt were spent, she got up from her father's grave and went home. But that wasn't the end of the story.

"A few days later," she told me, "I opened my mail and found a check for $3,000 from my father's brother. My uncle Clinton Whitney was dying of an incurable disease, so he was getting his house in order and liquidating his estate." The letter read:

> Dear Grace,
> Please think of this money as a gift from your father. It comes from my own estate, but I'm giving it to you in his name. I know he loved you, and he was always proud of you.
> Please divide this money as follows: Give $1,000 to each of your sons, and keep $1,000 for yourself.
> With love,
>
> Clinton Whitney

"My uncle sent that letter," Grace told me, "on the very day I was at the cemetery, making amends to my father. It was as if my father had sent me the check himself to tell me, 'Grace, I heard everything you said, and all is forgiven—and just to show you I love you, here's a little bonus! Enjoy!'"

Grace Lee Whitney found life after guilt, and so can you. Guilt is a wake-up call, not a death knell. Listen to your guilt feelings, learn from them, grow from them. Then put your life in order and *live*.

Questioning Life

11

How Can I Find Happiness?

The English philosopher Bertrand Russell was sitting in his garden, a pensive expression on his face, when a friend happened by. "Why so thoughtful?" asked the friend.

For a few seconds, Russell seemed not to have heard the question. Then he shook himself from his reverie. "Eh? Oh. I've just made the most fascinating discovery. Every time I talk to a learned scholar, I am convinced that it is impossible to be happy in life. But when I talk to my gardener, I am forced to the opposite conclusion."

Bertrand Russell's gardener knew. Happiness is not reserved for the learned or the rich or the winners of life's lottery. Some of the happiest people in this world are the simplest, most common of people, and even people who have endured great hardship and suffering. Paradoxically, I've noticed that some of the richest, most highly achieving people are the least happy.

So where does happiness come from? And how can we find it?

You don't get it by pursuing it

It's as American as the Declaration of Independence: We have a right to "life, liberty and the pursuit of happiness." In fact, it seems that everywhere we turn in America, we are not just given the *right* to be happy, we are practically *ordered* to be happy—as in the words of that stupid Bobby McFerrin song, "Don't worry: be happy!"

Psychologist Viktor Frankl, the Auschwitz survivor and originator of logotherapy, once observed, "Happiness cannot be pursued; it must ensue."[1] In other words, in order to be happy, we must not make happiness our goal. Happiness only comes as the by-product of pursuing something *other* than happiness. But what? If we can't be happy by pursuing happiness, what should we pursue instead? Answer: We must pursue a *reason* to be happy.

Frankl used this analogy: Tell a man to laugh, and if he does, it will probably sound hollow and forced. But tell him a really good joke, and he'll laugh. Why? Because you've given him a *reason* to laugh. It's the same with happiness. Tell a grumpy man, "Be happy," and you'll probably just make him grumpier. It's not enough to *want* to be happy. You've got to have a *reason* to be happy. If you have a reason, then happiness naturally ensues.

So what is a good reason for being happy? Some people would say prosperity brings happiness. Others say pleasure brings happiness. Well, our nation has never been more prosperous, and we've never had more pleasures to spend our prosperity on—but, seemingly, we've never been less happy. If we are happy, why are drug abuse and alcohol abuse so rampant in our society? Why do an average of eighty-six Americans commit suicide every day?[2]

I would submit to you that one major reason for all this unhappiness is that life for most people today is meaningless. Money doesn't make life meaningful. Neither does pleasure. Neither does sex or status or power or any of the other things we chase after. When people live meaningless lives, they respond with depression, aggression, and addiction. Depression is sometimes acted out by self-destruction (suicide); aggression is often played out through acts of destruction (crime and other antisocial behavior); addiction is the result of trying to numb the pain of meaninglessness with alcohol, drugs, or other compulsive behavior.

In order to be happy, our goal should not be happiness, but *completeness*. When we are complete people, our lives have meaning, and our souls experience that sense of satisfaction and peace that produces *true* happiness.

Seven principles for a happy life

Happiness is no accident, no stroke of good fortune. Happiness is a *choice*. The kind of people we are is determined by the decisions and choices we make, the attitude we adopt. No matter what life does to us, inflicts on us, or takes away from us, we always have the freedom to choose how we will respond.

So how do we choose an attitude of happiness? Here are some practical principles for a happy life:

Happiness Principle No. 1: Take responsibility for your own life and your own happiness.

If you're unhappy, stop blaming other people or God or bad luck for your unhappiness. Accept responsibility for your life. As long as we put the blame elsewhere, we feel helpless and trapped. But when we accept the responsibility for our own happiness, we feel empowered to make changes that lead to true happiness and satisfaction in life.

Understand that moods and emotions (including happiness and unhappiness) are temporary. If you are unhappy now, you probably feel engulfed by it. Your unhappiness feels like a permanent condition—but it's not. If you look at your moods objectively and rationally, you realize that moods come and go. Happiness is temporary, but so is unhappiness.

If your moods go up and down, it can be helpful to keep a journal. Write down your feelings and experiences (that's called "externalizing"). It often helps to take those feelings out of your mind and soul, and set them down on paper. Write down everything that comes to mind that relates to how you feel, both when you are up and when you are down. Journaling accomplishes two important functions:

First, journaling is a good way to bleed off emotional poisons. Write everything down without editing; let your stream of consciousness flow into your journal. The emotional catharsis can often do you a world of good.

Second, journaling gives you a record of your good moods. When you are unhappy, go back and read the happy portions of your journal. This will help restore a balanced perspective. You'll be able to see that the unhappy periods in your life are temporary, and you'll be able to reread and relive the happy times.

Happiness Principle No. 2: Tune in to your feelings and motives.

Tuning in to your moods, emotions, and motivations is a lot like tuning in a station on the radio. Sometimes you have to twiddle the dial until the reception improves. From time to time, we need to pay close attention to what we are thinking and feeling, so we can make adjustments. Our surface motives are not always the motives that truly drive our feelings and behavior.

Some people actually cling to their unhappiness because, on some hidden and unhealthy level, they *gain* something from being unhappy. Moping and sulking can become a tool for manipulating family members, getting your way, attracting attention, or punishing others. This is one of the ways we choose to stay in an unhealthy place. We *think* we want to be happy, we *say* we want to be happy, yet we continually *choose* to be unhappy in order to get something we want. As we become more aware of our true motivations and the reasons for our unhealthy behavior, we can begin to make healthier, happier choices.

Severe unhappiness or depression can be a warning sign that something is out of whack in your life. It could be a warning sign from your body of a physical problem that needs to be addressed. It could be a warning sign of problems in your relationships, your career, or your mental health.

If your depression lasts more than a week or two—and particularly if you begin experiencing destructive or self-destructive thoughts—you should have an immediate physical checkup by your doctor or a consultation with a professional psychologist or psychiatrist. There's a difference between a temporary bout of unhappiness (which may be triggered by specific problems and circumstances, such as a loss or setback in life) and clinical depression, which requires professional intervention.

People with a temporary bout of unhappiness can usually express their feelings in a realistic way. According to psychologist Dr. James Osterhaus, clinical depression may involve more vague and generalized feelings of sadness, anger, guilt, fatigue, restlessness, listlessness, hopelessness, and worthlessness. A person with clinical depression may have thoughts of death or self-destruction, loss of appetite and interest in pleasurable activities, changes in weight or appetite, changes in sleep patterns, and an inability to remember, concentrate, and make decisions. If you experience some of these symptoms, don't try to solve your depression by reading a book—see your doctor right away.

Happiness Principle No. 3: Focus on others instead of self.

Unhappy people are focused on themselves. Happy people are focused on others. The most cheerful and contented people I know are those who are involved in volunteering, taking in foreign exchange students, tutoring students, visiting shut-ins, and otherwise involving themselves in meeting the needs of others.

Happy people go out of their way to make friends—and shyness is no excuse for not making friends. As I noted in a previous chapter, I'm a shy person myself. But one day it hit me

> "*H*appy people are focused on others."

that shyness is really a form of pride. Shyness puts the focus onto yourself instead of others. The person who says, "I'm shy," is really saying, "What will people think of me?" Ever notice how the words "painful" and "shy" go together, as in the phrase, "She's painfully shy"? I don't know any seriously shy people who are really happy. Why? Because they are focused on themselves instead of others.

If you want to make friends, it's easy. Just stop thinking about yourself, and start thinking about others. Find out what other people are interested in, what they like, what makes them tick. Look people in the eye. Smile. Don't force it, but be naturally friendly and interested in others. Instead of talking about yourself, ask questions and get the other person to talk about himself or herself. Make the other person feel important. Focus on others instead of yourself, and you're guaranteed to make friends.

Happiness Principle No. 4: Get rid of poisonous emotions.

Feelings of anger, bitterness, and guilt are destructive to your happiness, so do everything you can to resolve conflicts in your most important relationships. Let go of grudges. When the other person is wrong, resolve it and forgive. When you are wrong, apologize and be forgiven. Unhappiness results whenever we focus on punishing others or punishing ourselves with guilt. Put wrongs in the past where they belong; don't keep them in the present where they gnaw on you and destroy your happiness.

Happiness Principle No. 5: Make time for simple pleasures.

Sometimes the simplest and smallest of luxuries and rewards can make you feel as happy as if you just hit the lottery. Think of how good you feel when you take that first sip of a perfect cup of coffee. Or when you bite into a chocolate, thinking it's probably filled with that disgusting brandied fruit stuff, and it turns out to be your favorite creme filling. Or when your insurance company sends you a dividend check for $37.42.

Or when you just sit on the back porch with your family and watch the most perfect sunset you've ever seen.

Even in tough times, we can find happiness in the small pleasures and simple joys of life. So treat yourself to a simple pleasure. Take time to savor life and enjoy pleasurable moments. When you can't find happiness in the big stuff, take refuge in the little stuff. Instead of focusing where the happiness isn't, focus on where it is.

Happiness Principle No. 6: Change the thinking and behavior that produces unhappiness.

You can't always control how you feel, but you can control what you think and do. Our feelings are generally determined by our thoughts and behavior. In fact, *feelings follow thoughts* and *feelings follow behavior*. To be happy, think the thoughts of a happy person and do the actions of a happy person—and your feelings will naturally follow.

What have you been thinking about that makes you unhappy? Such thoughts usually have to do with anger ("How could she do that to me!"), bitterness ("I'll never forgive and I'll never forget!"), hopelessness ("This is my lot in life and it will never change"), self-hate ("I always do the wrong thing! Why am I so stupid?"), and so forth. To become a happy person, you have to make a deliberate, conscious decision to think the thoughts of a happy person—thoughts of understanding ("There must be some reason she acted that way"), forgiveness ("I won't let this memory eat me up inside—I choose to let go of it"), hope ("I have the power to make my life better—and I will"), and self-acceptance ("A mistake's not so bad—I'm going to learn and grow from this").

Unhappy people usually engage in behavior that reinforces and worsens their unhappiness, so one of the keys to changing your mood is changing your behavior. The behaviors that help to lift your mood include:

- laughing—watch a sitcom or stand-up comedy show on TV, rent a comedy video, get together with friends who make you laugh;

- exercising—get out and take a walk, go to the gym, take up a sport;

- eating right—be aware of foods that alter your moods, such as sugar, caffeine, and alcohol;

- maintaining a regular routine—get the right amount of sleep but avoid lying in bed thinking unhappy thoughts; establish a daily schedule of pursuing your goals and stick to it;

- cleaning house—a messy environment is depressing; a tidy environment lifts your mood.

Happiness Principle No. 7: Stop comparing yourself with others; replace envy with thankfulness.

There's no point wishing you could trade places with someone else. Everybody has struggles. Some people, for example, would no doubt envy the beauty of a supermodel, and think, "I wish I'd been born beautiful like her—then everything would come easy for me like it does for her." Yet supermodel Kim Alexis told me that, as a teenager, she considered her appearance a drawback.

"I felt punished for being beautiful," she told me. "The kids at school avoided me. I once asked my dad why that was, and he said, 'Honey, it's because you're beautiful. The boys won't ask you out because they're afraid you'll say no. Teenage boys would rather not ask you out than risk rejection.' I thought that was so unfair! I said, 'But I don't want to be beautiful! I just want to be popular!' People think being beautiful is a free ticket to happiness, but it's not. Everybody has insecurities and problems. I've found that the key to satisfaction is to stop envying others and to be content with what you have."

Some of the happiest people I know have little in the way of beauty, fame, or possessions. And some of the most miserable people I know are those who have done quite well in life—*yet they have little appreciation for their good fortune*. Why? Because they are busily comparing themselves with others who have even *more* (or so they think).

It has been said that it is better to win a bronze medal in the Olympics than the silver. Why? Comparisons! The silver winner groans inwardly, *Arrgghh! I came THIS CLOSE to winning the gold!* That's an attitude of envy. The bronze winner, however, is pleased with her good fortune: *How lucky! I came THIS CLOSE to not winning anything!* That's an attitude of thankfulness.

A happy person is a thankful person. Gratitude and envy cannot coexist in a human soul. One or the other must rule. So if your mind and soul are ruled by an attitude of thankfulness, then envy and the resulting unhappiness will not be able to gain a foothold in your life. As G. K. Chesterton once observed, "There are two ways to get enough. One is to continue to accumulate more and more. The other is to be content with less."

You have the key

The most mistaken notion most of us have about happiness is thinking that our happiness depends on our circumstances. We suppose, "If I had only married the right person—" or, "If I just made more money—" or, "If my parents hadn't been so abusive when I was a kid, then I could be happy right now." Wrong. Fact is, happiness doesn't come from our circumstances but from the way we think about our circumstances.

During the lean, tough years of my early writing career, a friend gave me a slim, 164-page book, *The Choice* by Og Mandino. She said the book had meant a lot to her during some trying times, and she thought it might be helpful to me. I knew that Og Mandino was a motivational writer in the Napoleon Hill/Maxwell Maltz/Zig Ziglar mold, and most of my life I had not seen much point in reading motivational writers. But with the career struggles I was going through at the time, I was ripe for this book. I opened it and on the first page I found this quotation by Charles Fletcher Lummis:

> I am bigger than anything that can happen to me. All these things—sorrow, misfortune, and suffering—are outside my door. I am in the house and I have the key.

That statement hit me right between the eyes—and so did the rest of the book. I won't go into detail about the content of the book. I'll just say that Mandino's central theme is that we all have the power to choose how we will live our lives, regardless of our circumstances. Few of us really understand and appreciate this amazing power to choose our attitude. Instead, we wallow in self-pity and unhappiness, thinking our lives are shaped for us by fate, circumstances, and outside forces. In reality, our lives are primarily shaped by our own thoughts, attitudes, and choices. As Abraham Lincoln observed, "Most people are about as happy as they make up their minds to be."

The message of *The Choice* was just what I needed at that time. My circumstances were bleak—I was in debt, my bank account was empty, I had a mortgage to pay and a family to support, and my next paycheck was weeks away. But in order to collect that paycheck, I had to finish the book I was writing—and to do that, I needed to stay positive, energized, and upbeat. Nothing dries up a writer's muse like worry, stress, and depression. Reading *The Choice* was one factor that got me through those tough times.

Though his book had a powerful influence on me at a crucial time in my life, I have never met Og Mandino—but a friend of mine has. In the summer of 1996, Pat Williams, executive vice president of the Orlando Magic organization, phoned me, very excited. "Jimbo," he said (Pat's the only person who's allowed to call me that!), "you'll never guess who I met yesterday." Well, Pat seems to be on a first-name basis with everybody who is anybody, so I couldn't guess. "I met one of my heroes," he continued, "Og Mandino."

It turned out that Pat and Og had shared a podium at the National Speakers Association convention in Orlando. Before speaking, Pat chatted with Og Mandino about his book *Secrets for Success and Happiness.* Mandino thanked Pat for his compliments on the book, then added, "Let me tell you something about that book. I haven't seen my daughter in forty-two years. When she was little, I had an alcohol problem. I loved my daughter and wanted to be a good father, but my drinking got in the way. My wife divorced me and took my daughter away and I haven't seen either one of them since. I can't imagine what my ex-wife told my little girl about me, but it must have been horrible enough to keep her from wanting any contact for more than four decades. But just six months ago, I got a letter from my daughter. She had bought that book and read it— and then she called me to seek a reconciliation. We haven't seen each other yet, but we're exchanging letters. We both want to let go of the past and find each other again."

It was just six weeks after that conversation that seventy-three-year-old Og Mandino fell and struck his head. He was found dead the following morning. Did Og Mandino and his daughter ever get together for that hoped-for reunion? I don't know. But at least a door had been opened and they were reaching out to each other.

It's hard for me to imagine the pain of being separated from a child for decades. Yet throughout those decades, Og Mandino made a choice not to be a prisoner of his past and his circumstances. He made a choice to be happy. He lived out the philosophy that Sara Teasdale affirmed when she wrote, "I make the most of all that comes and the least of all that goes." What's more, through his many books and countless speaking appearances, he preached the truth to millions that *happiness is a choice*.

Happiness is a choice that *you* can make as well. You are bigger than anything that can happen to you. Sorrow, misfortune, and suffering are all outside your door and beyond your walls. You are in the house, and you have the key.

What Is Truth?

Kathy Myatt is a registered nurse and mental health specialist in Rio de Janeiro. She recalls a patient she encountered while working in a psychiatric hospital in Colorado. The patient was admitted to the hospital claiming to be Jesus Christ. The doctor prescribed a powerful psychotropic medication, Haldol (haloperidol). After a few doses, the man backed down from his claim to be Jesus, and instead claimed to be the "fourth member of the Trinity"—apparently unaware of the numerical paradox that claim implied. A few more doses of Haldol, and the patient revised his claim once more—now he was "one of the Beatles."

Finally, after a week of antipsychotic treatment, the man was asked who he was—and he gave his right name and identity. With continued treatment, he was able to return to his family and resume his life and career.

What had happened to this man? He had experienced a serious psychotic episode due, at least in part, to an imbalance in his brain chemistry (*psychotic* means to be afflicted with a severe mental disorder that involves losing contact with reality). With medical help, the man's mental balance was restored—and so was his grip on objective reality. He was once again able to grasp the truth about himself and the world around him.

After relating this story, Kathy Myatt asks a crucial question: Since the underlying assumption in our culture today is that "truth" is merely a matter of personal perception, personal preference, and subjective experience, why medicate the man? After all, we are increasingly told today that there is no such thing as objective truth. So why not let him go on believing he is Jesus Christ? "What if he was right?" asks Myatt. "Who were we to say that he was indeed *not* Jesus Christ—or one of the Beatles? Why did we not simply bow down and worship him? Or beg him to play a song?"[1]

These are important questions. There is a refrain I hear all the time, and perhaps you do, too: "You have your truth. I have my truth. There's no such thing as *true* truth." So is truth really important? More to the point: Is there even such a thing as truth?

Where has truth gone?

Many people today are unaware of the profound shift in thinking that has taken place in recent decades. Near the beginning of the twentieth century, for example, Einstein's theory of relativity upset the old Newtonian assumptions about the nature of reality. One of the implications of Einstein's theory is that space and time—which once were thought to be fixed and absolute—are *relative* concepts. Space is curved by gravity, and the rate at which time passes is affected by gravity and velocity.

As often happens with scientific subjects, the implications of Einstein's theory have been widely misreported in the media and widely misunderstood by the public. As information about Einstein's theory trickled into the public consciousness, a misimpression formed: If space and time are no longer absolute, then there are no absolutes. If there are no absolutes, then there is no such thing as absolute (or objective) truth.

The name of Einstein's theory—*relativity*—didn't help matters. From a misunderstanding of relativity came a concept called *relativism*—the belief that conceptions of truth and reality are purely subjective. In a world of relativism, "truth" is nothing more than an opinion, and no opinion is more or less valid than any other opinion. When everything is relative, nothing is *true*.

The result is that we now have an entire culture that has been saturated with the notion that "everything is relative." Most people even have some vague notion that Einstein *proved* that "everything is relative." Einstein, however, proved nothing of the sort. There definitely are absolutes in Einstein's picture of reality (the invariable value of c, the speed of light, is a prime example). Einstein himself often referred to his concept as "invariance theory," because it demonstrated the fact that physical laws remain constant and absolute—they do not vary—regardless of one's frame of reference. So not only does Einstein's theory *not* support relativism, it specifically contradicts it.

The cultural relativism that came from a misreading of Einstein's theory was not a total disaster. Relativism gave us nonobjective art (such as the cubists—Picasso, Georges Braque, Marcel Duchamp); the nonobjective poetry of T. S. Eliot ("For last year's words belong to last year's language / And next year's words await another voice"); and the nonobjective fiction of James Joyce ("All things are inconstant except the faith in the soul"). There is a joyous chaoticism in the art of relativism.

But the achievements of relativism in the arts are more than overshadowed by relativism's dark side. As a political and social philosophy, relativism has caused untold human misery. Where there is no objective truth, there is no objective morality. Concepts like human freedom, human dignity, and human rights are no longer considered absolute truths in a world of relativism. They are just words. From the moral and social relativism of Karl Marx, we get Lenin, Stalin, the purges, and the gulags. Hitler, too, was spawned in a climate of moral relativism. So were the killers at Columbine High School. In a world where nothing is right anymore, nothing is wrong, either—not even mass murder.

Ultimately, relativism trickles down, saturating the consciousness of the masses through books, films, and television. It has infected the minds of the coming generation through our educational system. As a result, many young people today have little use for logical arguments—not because these kids are stupid or lazy, but because there are too many conflicting viewpoints to deal with. It's too chaotic, too confusing. So they survive in a confusing world by focusing on relationships, emotions, and what *feels* good—not what's objectively true. My truth and your truth are equally valid, even if they utterly conflict—*and many people today see no contradiction in that view.*

A disturbing example of this trend is offered by Professor Robert Simon, who teaches at Hamilton College in New York State. He observes that increasing numbers of students no longer acknowledge that the Holocaust—the systematic liquidation of six million human beings—was morally wrong. While his students say they *personally* find mass murder to be disagreeable, as many as 20 percent of his students express their disapproval only as a "personal preference." Said one student, "Of course I dislike the Nazis, but who is to say they are morally wrong?"[2]

Christina Hoff Sommers, professor of philosophy at Clark University, says she has tried and failed to find any crime, any atrocity, that her first-year students might condemn as morally intolerable. Would it be objectively wrong to torture a child? To starve someone to death? To abuse and humiliate an invalid in a nursing home? The reply of her students: "Torture, starvation, and humiliation may be bad for you or for me, but who are we to say they are bad for someone else?" Concludes Thomas Lickona, professor of education at the State University of New York at Cortland:

> Students' moral relativism, of course, is just one expression of subjectivism—the intellectual belief that all truth is subjective. Boston College philosopher Peter Kreeft calls this "a crisis of truth." "Of all the symptoms of decay in our decadent civilization," he says, "subjectivism is the most disastrous of all. A mistake—be it a moral mistake or an intellectual mistake—can be discovered and corrected only if truth exists and can be known."[3]

I encountered the same attitudes while posting on a couple of Internet bulletin board services, called BBSs for short. I began by posting a topic—or "thread"—that had to do with the question of objective truth. The topic generated numerous posts (messages) from people around the world, most of them roughly college age. More than half were up-front about the fact that they did not believe in objective truth or absolute right and wrong. When I cited the Nazi Holocaust and the Columbine massacre as examples of absolute evil, many refused to call these events "evil" or "wrong." A sampling of their responses:

- "There is no such thing as evil, only a perception of evil."

- "People don't set out to do evil—those kids [the Columbine killers] probably thought they were doing a good thing."

- "Good and evil, by their very nature, are subjective. What's evil to one person isn't necessarily evil to everyone else. There is no real evil—just a bunch of opinions."

- "Evil is subjective. Morality is relative. Next to my interests, the interests of my fellow man are irrelevant."

I had a fascinating online discussion with the young man who posted that last statement. I wrote, "You say 'Evil is subjective' with such *objective* finality. How do you *objectively* know that evil is subjective? ;-)" He replied that it didn't matter if it was objectively true. Why? "Because," he wrote, "as far as I'm concerned, I'm all there is. I cannot prove that god, or even you, exist. So I'm all that matters, and to heck with everyone else." I pointed out that this was an old idea called *solipsism*—the belief that one's own self is the only reality. My parting shot was, "Something for you to think about—assuming, of course, that *you* exist. ;-)" His reply: "I was disappointed when I learned a few months ago from my history teacher that I wasn't the first with this perspective. He called solipsism the 'quintessential teenage philosophy.' But don't worry about *me* existing, it's *you* I'm worried about. ;-)"

It was a cordial exchange—but chilling nonetheless. My discussions on that Internet BBS demonstrated how deeply entrenched the mindset of relativism has become. More than once in these discussions, I've seen that slogan parroted: "Everything is relative." But everything is *not* relative. Truth is *not* a matter of opinion. Truth is what is *real* regardless of opinion, regardless of whether anyone believes it or not.

Example: For most of human history, people thought the Earth was flat, and that it was the center of the universe. But human opinion was *wrong*. For some four and a half billion years, Planet Earth has been a ball-shaped world circling a star that happened to be plodding around the outskirts of the Milky Way galaxy—hardly the center of the universe. The fact that no one was aware of this truth did not make it any less true. Truth is completely independent of human opinion.

You have your opinion, I have mine, but *truth*—real, objective, *true* truth—has a reality all its own.

Deconstructing truth

The Spring/Summer 1996 issue of *Social Text*, an American journal of cultural studies, heralded an article with the title, "Transgressing the Boundaries: Towards a Transformative Hermeneutics of Quantum Gravity." Certainly sounds impressive, doesn't it?

The article, written by physicist Alan Sokal of New York University, claimed to expose the corrupt philosophical and political underpinnings of quantum physics. Sokal attacked Western physicists for promoting a "dogma imposed by the long post-Enlightenment hegemony over the Western intellectual outlook" regarding the existence of an "external world, whose properties are independent of any individual human beings." Translation: Physicists are falsely promoting belief in objective reality.

Sokal went on to call for an "emancipatory mathematics" free of the taint of capitalism and Western thought. He proposed a "liberatory physics" that would emerge from the theory of quantum gravity. This new "liberatory physics," the author claimed, would ultimately prove the validity of liberal political ideology. Sokal's piece had all the standard accoutrements of an academic thesis, including plenty of incomprehensible jargon, lengthy quotes, and scholarly footnotes.

Once his paper had been published in *Social Text*, Sokal then published a second paper, this time in the journal *Lingua Franca*. There, he made an announcement that rocked the intellectual community: The paper in *Social Text* was a hoax—and a test. He wanted to see if the editors at *Social Text* had become so ideologically biased and intellectually lazy that they would publish a hodgepodge of ridiculous assertions, mathematical and scientific absurdities, and arcane quotations, believing it to be a serious academic paper. Sokal admitted using "the silliest quotations about math and physics I could find from prominent French and American intellectuals." The editors had taken the bait, and Sokal had reeled them in. The purpose of the hoax, he said, was to expose "the postmodern abuse of science."[4]

And here we get to the nub of Sokal's grudge: A worldview called *postmodernism*, which has massively infected academic thinking. Postmodernism has immersed an entire generation in the belief that there is no such thing as objective truth. As social critic Kenan Malik observes in *New Statesman*:

> The real target of [Sokal's] critique is not so much the nonsensical jargon of postmodernism as its relentless relativism—the view that scientific knowledge is not universal, but the product of particular social and cultural circumstances. Sokal challenges the idea that the modern physicist's view of nature is no more or less valid than that of the Australian Aborigine or the American Creationist.[5]

Postmodernism is an assault upon the concept of objective truth. It is the academic equivalent of the popular slogan, "Everything is relative." The "modernism" that postmodernism attempts to supplant began with the Enlightenment in the eighteenth century. The leaders of the Age of Enlightenment believed that, through the application of rational principles and the acquisition of knowledge, they could usher in a Utopia. One of the fundamental assumptions of the Enlightenment was the belief that the external world was real, accessible to our senses, and knowable, as this statement by Voltaire demonstrates:

> This is the character of truth: It is of all time, it is for all men, it has only to show itself to be recognized, and one cannot argue against it.

Postmodernism would damn Voltaire as a deluded fool. To the postmodernist, truth is not something that is discovered and recognized— it is something we invent.

The centerpiece of postmodernism is *deconstructionism*. First proposed by the arch-postmodern philosopher Jacques Derrida in the 1970s, deconstructionism was originally a theory about language and literature that claimed that words have no objective content. *Deconstruction* comes from the merger of the words *destruction* and *construction*. Derrida's goal was to deconstruct language, to turn words upside-down and drain them of objective content. Today, deconstructionism has pervaded many areas of human endeavor: academia, feminism, sociology, theology, journalism, law, and, politics (where the fate of a president once hinged on what the meaning of "is" is). Those who believe reality can be comprehended by language, so as to yield "truth," suffer from "radical delusion," say the deconstructionists.

Derrida claims that cultural conditioning and language structure shape the way we perceive reality. This view, however, ignores the large body of research showing that we do not primarily use words to process reality. We think at a nonverbal level, and then express those thoughts in words so that we can communicate them to other people. Derrida also ignores the fact that much of the language of science is mathematics—a "language" that is utterly precise and devoid of cultural bias. It is an objective fact that $2 + 2 = 4$, no matter what your cultural conditioning.

Deconstructionism scorns Western thinking for its "logocentrism," the notion that words can correspond to objective reality. From the postmodern point of view, there is no truth, no logic, no meaning, no objective reality.

The deconstructionists question everything—but I question the questioners. They say truth is unknowable; I say, "How do you *know* that to be true?" They say there are no absolutes; I say, "Are you *absolutely* sure?" Deconstructionism is inherently self-contradictory—and self- contradiction is proof that an idea is false—

At least in a rational world.

Truth and trust

Why does objective truth matter? For one thing, if you don't believe in truth, you might as well close this book and put it on a shelf. The chapters that follow will deal in verifiable evidence and objective fact. We're going to talk about God and the soul and related matters—but we're not going to deal in opinions or speculations. We're going to deal in facts and evidence. So if you don't believe in the reality of truth, we'll have nothing to discuss.

But there's yet another simple, basic reason why objective truth matters: Without *truth*, there can be no *trust*.

How can you trust someone who believes that truth is relative? A person who doesn't believe in truth doesn't believe in lies. And a person who doesn't believe in lies feels free to make up any "reality" he or she chooses. If you do not believe in objective truth, then "truth" can be anything you want it to be at any given moment. You can lie, and for you it will be your "truth," simply because you want it to be so.

How can society function without truth and trust? How can contracts and agreements have any meaning? How can laws have any meaning—including our ultimate law in America, the Constitution—without a common belief in objective truth? How can something as simple as a friendship be possible without the trust that is rooted in truth? If you are going to be my friend, I have to know I can trust you—and there is no trust without truth.

Business guru Harvey Mackay tells the story of a Duke University chemistry professor named Professor Bonk (his course was widely known as "Bonkistry"). One time, as finals week approached, two of Professor Bonk's male students were so confident of their straight-A averages that they decided to drive up to the University of Virginia to party with friends, confident that they could ace Monday's final exam.

They partied hard over the weekend. Sunday morning found them nursing the worst hangovers of their lives. In fact, they were so sick, they didn't start back for the Duke campus until early Monday morning, the day of the test.

They arrived at Professor Bonk's room a few minutes before class and gave him a story that was part truth—and part "deconstructed truth." They said, "Professor, we were planning to be back from Virginia in time to study, but on the way we got a flat tire. We didn't have a spare, and it took hours to fix, so we didn't get back to the dorm until late last night. By then it was too late to study."

Professor Bonk considered their story—then agreed to let them make up the test the following day. The two young men breathed a sigh of relief, then went back to the dorm to study.

The next morning, Professor Bonk put the two students in separate rooms across the hall from each other, each with a copy of the test booklet. From the hall, he checked his watch and said, "Begin." Then he closed the doors of the two rooms.

In seclusion, each student opened his test booklet. On the first page was a simple problem about molarity and solutions. The problem was worth five points. "Cool!" each young man said to himself. "This'll be a cinch!" It only took a couple minutes to answer the problem, and turn the page—

Gulp! The next page had just one question—the only other question on the exam: "Which tire? (95 points)."[6]

Truth is not relative. There is no pluralism of truths, no "your truth," no "my truth." There is only *true* truth—and that truth is reality itself.

What Is the Meaning of Life?

I was sixteen years old in the fall of 1969. I didn't think too deeply about the meaning of life in those days. I was too busy having fun, hanging out with my friends, expanding my collection of Marvel Comics, working out with the track team after school, and doing just enough homework to maintain a precarious B-minus average.

The meaning of life? Who cares! Life is fun. I'm gonna live forever. Someday I'm gonna be a famous writer, make a lot of money, and have even *more* fun than I'm having now. Isn't that meaning enough?

But in the fall of 1969, my world was rocked by a white-haired gentleman with a Viennese accent. His name was Viktor Frankl.

I was just one of five hundred students who sat in a room on a university campus and heard him give a talk. But his words, so softly spoken, invaded my soul with all the power of a thunderclap.

Never before or since, to my knowledge, have I been in the presence of a survivor of the Nazi death camps. Even as a shallow and self-centered teenager, I knew a lot about those camps. In our home was a six-volume set of photo books on World War II, and I had devoured those books from cover to cover. The final volume contained numerous photos of the liberated camps, and I never got over the sight of those skeletal survivors with their haunted, deep-socketed eyes; or the grisly crematoria with their doors open, with exposed skulls and naked rib cages protruding from mounds of ashes; or the mass graves filled with piles of emaciated corpses.

And here, before my eyes, was a man who had *been* there, who had *suffered* there, who had endured unimaginable horror, and who had triumphed over it all. Simply and quietly, without sensationalism or melodrama, Frankl described what life was like in Auschwitz and the three other Nazi death camps where he was held from 1942 to 1945.

And my outlook on life was forever changed.

An answer from heaven

Born in Vienna in 1905, Viktor Emil Frankl was the son of a Jewish official in the Austrian government. A Socialist in his youth, Frankl pursued a career in medicine and psychology. He spent several years working among suicide attemptees. In 1938, after Nazi Germany forcibly annexed Austria, he became director of the neurology department of Rothschild Hospital, the only Jewish hospital in the Third Reich. During those years, he formulated a new meaning-centered approach to psychological therapy called *logotherapy* (from *logos*, the Greek word for "meaning").

At the beginning of World War II, Frankl had a chance to escape the Holocaust. All around him, Jewish families were being rounded up, forced onto cattle trains, and shipped to concentration camps. Rumors were flying that these facilities were actually *extermination* camps. When the American consulate in Vienna offered Frankl a visa allowing him to emigrate to the United States, he was relieved. But Frankl hesitated, wondering how he could leave his mother and father to an uncertain fate under the Nazis. His book on logotherapy was nearly completed in manuscript form; if he could emigrate to America, he could publish his work and help many people. If he refused the visa, his work might be lost, his life might be lost, and he could do nothing to save his parents in any case. Still, he could not decide whether to stay or go.

He wished for an answer from heaven—and the answer came in the form of a broken piece of marble he noticed on a table at his father's home. "What is that stone?" Frankl asked his father.

"I found it," replied the father, "at the place where the Nazis burned down our synagogue. I picked it up and kept it because it is a piece of the marble wall on which the Ten Commandments were engraved."

Frankl picked it up and examined it. There was a gilded Hebrew letter inscribed upon it—a letter which stood for one of the Commandments. "Which of the Commandments is this one?" asked Frankl.

"'Honor your father and your mother,'" quoted the father, "'that your days may be long upon the land.'"

That was Frankl's answer. He would remain in Vienna.

Soon afterward, Frankl, his young wife, and his parents were deported to Theresienstadt prison near Prague. He was separated from them, and during the years 1942 to 1945, he moved through a succession of camps, including the infamous chamber of horrors called Auschwitz.

He described being loaded onto a train at Theresienstadt, one of fifteen hundred people packed eighty to a car, with only a few tiny slits to let in light and air, and a pile of urine-soaked straw at one end of the car for relieving oneself. The prisoners were told they were being sent to a forced labor assignment at a munitions factory. They traveled for several days and nights without the cars being opened. Finally, the train slowed, pulling into a station. Someone near the air slits looked out and gasped, "Auschwitz!" With that word, all hope died.

Stepping down from the train, Frankl saw the chimneys above the crematoriums belching flame and smoke. Frankl didn't yet know what that smoke meant, but he would soon find out. In his hands, he clutched the manuscript he had carefully guarded while a prisoner at Theresienstadt. Some of his fellow prisoners asked the SS guards if they could keep a wedding ring or a good-luck medal; Frankl asked only that he be allowed to keep his book.

"I must preserve this book at all costs," he said. "It is my life's work."

The guard mocked him with an obscenity.

Only then did Frankl realize the truth. Everything would be taken from him. *Everything*.

Ordered to strip, he dropped his clothes and his book—his life's work—onto the floor. That was the last he ever saw of it.

A slender thread of fate

In Auschwitz, Frankl's theories about human meaning were put to the test, deepened, and refined by fire. "My deep desire to write this manuscript anew," he later recalled, "helped me to survive the rigors of the camps I was in. For instance, when in a camp in Bavaria I fell ill with typhus fever, I jotted down on little scraps of paper many notes intended to enable me to rewrite the manuscript, should I live to the day of liberation. I am sure that this reconstruction of my lost manuscript in the dark barracks of a Bavarian concentration camp assisted me in overcoming the danger of cardiovascular collapse."[1]

Daily life in the camps, Frankl recalled, was a "hard fight for existence...an unrelenting struggle for daily bread and for life itself." Prisoners lived on a tiny daily ration of hard bread and watery soup. Most guards were unrelentingly brutal, but if a guard thought you were a particularly good worker, he might tell the man at the soup pot to dip the ladle to the bottom and scoop out a few peas as a reward.

The goal of each prisoner was to stay strong enough to be useful to the Nazi taskmasters. Though trained as a doctor, Frankl's only use to the Nazis was as a trench digger and railroad track layer. Only by working hard could he stay alive. A prisoner who became too sick or feeble to work was sent to the gas chambers.

Of those who went into the camps, only a pitifully small number survived. Those who died the soonest were those who had no hope, no reason to live. One of Frankl's friends in prison was a man who had been a well-known composer and musician before his confinement. One day, at the beginning of March 1945, he confided a strange dream to Frankl. In the dream, a voice offered to grant the man one wish. His wish was to know when the war would end. The voice told him the day of liberation would be March 30. The man believed his dream was true, and that the end of his suffering was only weeks away.

The days passed, and it became clear that the war would not end by March 30. On the 29th, Frankl's friend became ill, running a high fever. On the 30th, he became delirious and lapsed into unconsciousness. On the 31st, just one day after the date in his dream, *and just one month before Hitler committed suicide in a Berlin bunker*—Frankl's friend died, apparently of typhoid fever. But in reality, Frankl concluded, it was the loss of hope and purpose that killed him.

Frankl quotes Nietzsche: "He who has a *why* to live for can bear with almost any *how*." Viktor Frankl had a *why* to live for, and that *why* enabled him to survive the *how* of the Holocaust. He concluded:

> Woe to him who saw no more sense in his life, no aim, no purpose, and therefore no point in carrying on. He was soon lost. The typical reply with which such a man rejected all encouraging arguments was, "I have nothing to expect from life any more." What sort of answer can one give to that?
>
> What was really needed was a fundamental change in our attitude toward life. We had to learn ourselves and, furthermore,

we had to teach the despairing men, that *it did not really matter what we expected from life, but rather what life expected from us.*[2]

In April 1945, Frankl was assigned to medical duties, though he was given no medicines to dispense and only scraps of waste paper for bandages. His work consisted mostly of helplessly watching people die of starvation and fever.

One day, the order was given to evacuate the camp and burn the buildings. When the evacuation trucks failed to arrive, the guards shut the prisoners in the wooden barracks and closed the gates. It appeared the camp was to be burned to the ground—prisoners and all.

Just then, the gates were opened and a car arrived. A Red Cross delegate from Geneva stepped out of the car and announced that the prisoners were under his protection. Frankl and the other prisoners were let out of the barracks and photographed. They wanted to leave, but the Red Cross delegate said, "It's too dangerous. Stay here. The Red Cross is sending trucks and you will soon be free." So the prisoners celebrated.

A few hours later, the Nazi Schutzstaffel (or SS) arrived with trucks. The prisoners, said the SS, would be sent to Switzerland in exchange for German POWs. The SS officers were uncharacteristically friendly and told the prisoners they had nothing to fear. So the prisoners boarded the trucks. Frankl stood in line, eager to go to Switzerland and freedom. But when the last of the trucks pulled away, Frankl was left behind. He had just missed getting a spot on the truck.

Discouraged, he and a few other remaining prisoners went into a deserted guard room to sleep that night. Sometime after midnight, he and the other prisoners were awakened by gunfire. The battle front had reached the camp. At dawn, the camp guards raised a white flag, and the Allied forces came in and found a nearly empty camp.

Frankl later learned that the "lucky" prisoners who had boarded the SS trucks for Switzerland had been taken instead to a row of buildings a few miles away. They were locked inside and the buildings were torched. All died. Frankl had narrowly survived by *not* getting his wish to board the truck! On such a slender thread did his fate depend.

The meaning of life

The day I heard Viktor Frankl tell his story in his own words, I knew I was sitting in the presence of a great human soul. The next day, I went to the library and checked out a copy of his book, *Man's Search for Meaning*. I took it home and devoured it. It's not a long book—only about 150 pages. But the depth of that book is astounding. I've reread it a number of times since, and it continues to affect my life with each new reading.

The core of Frankl's message is his concept of *logotherapy* or meaning-centered therapy. Put simply, Frankl advocates treating psychological and emotional problems by helping people discover *meaning* in life. Most forms of psychotherapy are *self*-centered. The patient comes to the therapist, talks about his problems for an hour, and repeats this process week after week, year after year, until the therapist's house, car, and boat are paid for. In the process, the patient's self-centeredness is coddled and reinforced.

Logotherapy turns this process inside-out. Instead of being self-centered like other forms of psychotherapy, logotherapy seeks to dismantle the self-centeredness that makes people neurotic. Instead of getting people *into* themselves, it gets people *out* of themselves. As patients become meaning-focused instead of self-focused, they find healing.

The need for meaning in life, says Frankl, is the most basic motivational force in human nature. The "will to meaning" is more important than the Freudian "will to pleasure" or the Adlerian "will to power." The meaning of life is a deeply individual and personal matter. We must each find our own meaning. No one else can find it for us.

To have meaning in life is to have something to live for—and something to die for. If there is nothing in this world that you would give your life for, then your life has no meaning. Everyone eventually dies, so we ought to make both life and death count for something—something big, something meaningful. Living only for pleasure, for status, for fame, for power, for money, for the acquisition of stuff—that's all transitory and meaningless. When they put you into a velvet-lined box, drop you in a hole, and shovel dirt over your face, what will your life have meant?

Smoke in the wind

Long before he picked up a guitar and earned a few gold records, my friend Barry McGuire was a teenager living in the fishing town of San Pedro, on Los Angeles Harbor. As a boy, he was drawn by the lure of the sea. He went out on the fishing boats, pulling nets all night long, listening to the stories the men told, sharing their liquor and cigarettes. On those hauls, he had a lot of time to think about life.

"One night, I was out on the deck," Barry told me, "smoking a cigarette and thinking about life and death. I took one last drag on my cigarette, then flicked it into the sea. I saw the red glow of it disappear, and I thought about the fact that it was now just a piece of soggy debris in the water, yet the smoke from it was still there, filling my lungs. *Man, life is like that cigarette*, I thought. *You live a while, then you're flicked off into the dark abyss like a spent butt. Isn't there anything left when you die, like the smoke that's still in my lungs? Is my whole life just a puff of smoke in the wind?*"

A few years later, Barry got a job as a pipe fitter in a machine shop. One day after lunch, Charlie, an old man who worked in the shop, went to Barry and said, "I don't feel so good. Could you give me a ride home?"

"Sure, Charlie," said Barry. "Wait here."

So Barry went to the office and told the foreman he was taking Charlie home. But when he got back to the shop, he found Charlie on the floor, dead. He was gone, just like that, leaving only an empty husk behind. A few minutes later, as several workers lifted the body and carried it away, Barry looked at Charlie's workbench—and there was a cigarette, still sending up a thin curl of smoke.

"I thought, *Man, what is it all about?*" recalls Barry. "*What is life, this thing that comes into existence so mysteriously and leaves us so suddenly? Charlie's gone and his cigarette is still burning. What does it all mean?* It really grabbed my head at that time: the mystery of life and death, the idea that one minute you're here and the next minute you're not. You never know if the next breath you take is going to be your last, and you could die never knowing why you were born, or why you lived, or why you died. Things like that made me wonder what my life meant, and what it was all about."

Nothin' means nothin'

Like Barry, we all wonder from time to time. Even though we easily get completely caught up in the race for status, power, sex, and possessions, we soon find out that none of those things truly satisfies the soul. We have never been richer as a society—and we have never been more empty and restless. As Frankl observes, we have enough to live by but nothing to live for; we have the means but no meaning.

The grand causes of the Baby Boomer generation have crumbled to dust. The Age of Aquarius has given way to the Age of AIDS. The tie-dyed radicals who preached "Make Love, Not War" have grayed into politicians who bomb Third World aspirin factories. Meet the new boss; same as the old boss. Young people today look at their parents and see that the Stop the War generation lives only for bigger SUVs and fatter 401(k)s. Where's the meaning in that?

You see it in the eyes of the young—the skaters, the Goths, the stoners, the gangsters, and even the preps, jocks, and cheerleaders: *Nothin' means nothin.'* The result, observes Frankl, is a "mass neurotic syndrome so pervasive in the young generation" characterized by three symptoms: depression, aggression, and addiction.[3] Depression is acted out in the alarming rate of teen suicide in our society. Aggression is acted out in teen violence, from bullying in school corridors to the slaughter at Columbine High. Addiction is acted out in the frightening amounts of crystal meth and crack cocaine consumed every day, from our inner city projects to our gated communities.

People who know the meaning of their lives do not commit suicide; they do not stab or shoot other people; they do not fry their brains on drugs. People who know the meaning of life neither destroy nor self-destruct. They *love* life and they *live* life.

In his book *The Unconscious God*, Viktor Frankl cites studies that show that 90 percent of alcoholics and 100 percent of drug addicts suffer from "an abysmal feeling of meaninglessness." My friend, actress Grace Lee Whitney, affirms the validity of those statistics. She attributes her own history of alcoholism and addiction to a sense of meaninglessness and purposelessness in life—a feeling she describes as "a hole in the gut with the wind blowing through." In a desperate attempt to fill that hole, she plunged into every addiction imaginable: drinking binges, drug binges, sex binges, gambling binges, all interspersed with horrible bouts of suicidal depression.

"Ever since I took my first drink at age thirteen," she told me, "I used alcohol as an anesthetic against the pain of a meaningless life." Only when Grace discovered a Higher Power and a higher purpose for her life (which she found in a Twelve Step recovery meeting) was she able to overcome her multiple addictions.

Steps to meaning

A writer is, above all, an observer. Over the years, as I have worked with great people—men and women who live meaningful, purposeful lives—I've noticed that certain traits are universal among them. I've tried to apply these findings to my own life, and I want to pass them along to you. Here, as I have observed them, are the steps to living a meaningful life.

Step 1: Find something greater than yourself to believe in— then commit yourself to it.

"The greatest use of life," said William James, "is to spend it for something that will outlast it." Some would say that art, literature, and science are greater than ourselves—but I wonder. As important as these endeavors may be, are any of them greater and more lasting than a human soul? If the Earth, the stars, and the universe itself have a limited life span (even a billion years is not an eternity), then all human creations— our most beautiful works of music, our greatest works of art—will eventually be erased.

But is there an endpoint to the human soul? Later in this book, we will examine evidence that we live on after the death of the body. If the soul is truly immortal, then it is greater and more permanent than our books, music, art work, and other achievements. Awards are eventually forgotten. Scientific discoveries are superceded. So what, if anything, truly outlasts this life?

I've interviewed scores of people, from celebrities to psychiatrists, and I've found one common denominator among all who live satisfied, meaningful lives: They experience a daily connection with the presence that is variously called God or a Higher Power or some other name. Those who make that daily connection have clearly found something to focus their lives upon—something that outlasts life itself. They have a powerful and profound reason for getting up and tackling the challenges of each new day.

If you and I have a Maker, then there must have been a purpose for which we were made—a purpose that extends beyond the limited horizon of our understanding. If we want to have a purpose in life that is deeper, higher, and greater than this life, then we should align our lives with that infinite, eternal purpose. It seems to me that anything less than that would be the waste of a lifetime.

Life is a problem, and you must solve it. Life is a question, and you must answer it. Every human being on the planet only gets one life to live, and when it's over, it's over—so don't blow it. Don't drift through life. Make the most of your one and only irreplaceable life. Find your deepest, greatest, highest aim and aspiration—then *commit* yourself to it, body and soul. Find the mission you were put on this earth to serve—then *accomplish* that mission.

Step 2: Live for the future.

Those who survived the concentration camps, observed Viktor Frankl, were the ones who looked to the future. Frankl himself lived to rewrite his destroyed book. While digging trenches in the bitter cold, he imagined himself after the war, standing in a warm, well-lit lecture hall, speaking to an audience on the psychology of the concentration camps (amazingly, I was privileged to sit in a warm, well-lit lecture hall and witness the fulfillment of his wish). Frankl lived by faith in the future. The prisoner who lost faith in the future, said Frankl, would mentally and physically waste away.

The same is true of you and me. Our lives must point toward tomorrow or we are condemned to an aimless existence.

Step 3: Struggle to achieve meaningful goals.

Good mental health requires a healthy tension between what we have *already* accomplished and what we have *yet* to accomplish. Frankl called it "the gap between what one is and what one should become." As long as we strive to close that gap, we have a purpose for living. Human beings are not designed to live in tensionless homeostasis, of endless rounds of golf or lounging on the beach. We are happiest, most energized, and most truly alive when we are striving for a worthwhile goal.

The key word here is "worthwhile." The drive to find meaning in life is the most basic of human drives, but we easily mistake it for something else. We sense this drive as a restlessness, a yearning for completion and satisfaction, and we mistakenly suppose, "If only I had enough power, or fame, or money, or sexual pleasure, then I would be satisfied, my life would have meaning." Those who chase after such things are inevitably disappointed. You can never get enough to be satisfied. That's why the rich keep chasing more riches, and the sexually obsessed have libidos that are never satiated.

Step 4: Forget yourself.

Or, more precisely, forget your *self*. There was a time when people focused on nurturing the soul. Now they just gratify the self. The self is a mighty poor substitute for the soul. The key to finding true meaning and purpose in life lies in self-transcendence. The more we forget ourselves by serving a cause greater than ourselves, the more meaning and purpose we discover in our lives.

Step 5: Learn to love.

Love—love in all its forms—gives meaning to life. Love of God; love of fellow human beings; love of a husband, wife, children, or other family members; love of goodness, beauty, or truth; love for people in need, people who are suffering. We experience life in all its splendor through love.

Love enables us to understand the inner reality of another person to almost the same degree that we understand ourselves. Love enables us to forgive those who have wronged us. Love enables us to recognize the potential and possibilities in another person. Through love, we experience another person in all of his or her uniqueness—and that is a profoundly meaningful experience.

Step 6: Learn to find meaning in all of life—including suffering.

Suffering is a part of life. For those whose lives have no meaning, suffering is nothing but senseless torment, and death is nothing but the termination of a pointless existence. But when your life is full of meaning, you know that suffering is never wasted because it deepens character—and you know that your death will mark the completion of a life well-lived.

Our response to problems and sufferings determines whether or not we are *worthy* of our sufferings. When we suffer, we have a choice to remain dignified, courageous, and loving—or we can choose to become bitter, vengeful, and hateful, losing our human dignity in the process. When we cannot change our circumstances, we have to allow our circumstances to *change us*. We have to cooperate with our sufferings so that we can be made stronger, wiser, and more loving by our sufferings. If we meet our fate with dignity, courage, and love, then everything that happens to us, even death itself, has meaning.

Step 7: Live your life as a monument to the meaning you have chosen.

Life is short, but the brevity of life does not negate its meaning. The brevity of life simply tells us that we have no time to waste. Life's shortness intensifies its sweetness. Now is the hour. The opportunities to make our lives count are before us today. Tomorrow may be too late. So we need to make sure we spend our brief span of life on the things that are greater than ourselves. Are you only leaving behind footprints on a shifting sand dune—or are you leaving behind a lasting monument to something greater than yourself? When you are gone, will it matter to the world that you once lived?

Steven Spielberg's motion picture *Schindler's List* has a lot to teach us about the meaning of life. It is the story of Oskar Schindler, a businessman in Krakow, Poland, during the Holocaust in World War II. Schindler is a complex man who lusts for money, power, and women, yet he also develops a heart of compassion for the Jews who work as slave laborers in his factory. At enormous cost to himself, Schindler saves many Jews, purchasing their lives and saving them from extermination.

There is a scene near the end of the film in which Oskar Schindler (Liam Neeson) is surrounded by hundreds of people—the Jewish men and women he has saved from extermination in the death camps. A spokesman for the Jews, Itzhak Stern (Ben Kingsley) steps forward and presents Schindler with a letter of gratitude signed by everyone present. Then Stern hands Schindler a gold ring inscribed with these words from the Hebrew Talmud: "Whoever saves one life saves the world entire."

Schindler is moved and nearly speechless—not so much by their own gratitude as by his own guilt and regret. "I—I could have gotten more out," he confesses, his face filled with anguish. "I could have gotten more, if I just—I could have gotten more—"

"Oskar," says Stern, "there are eleven hundred people alive because of you. Look at them."

Schindler refuses to be comforted. "If I'd made more money—I threw away so much money! You have no idea—"

"There will be generations because of what you did," Stern insists.

"I didn't do enough!"

"You did so much."

Schindler puts his hands on his sleek black limousine. "This car—"

he moans. "Why did I keep this car? I could have sold it and bought ten more people." He removes his lapel pin and looks at it with disgust. "This pin! This is gold! It would have bought two more people!" He collapses in tears. "I could have gotten more people, and I didn't! I didn't—"

Later, as he is driven away in the back of his limousine, he looks out the window of the car. We see his anguished face reflected in the glass, and beyond the window pass the faces of people he has saved. But he can't see the ones he has saved. As the faces parade past, they seem to be the faces of those he could have saved, but didn't. Those faces haunt him....

What is the meaning of your life? Are you using your life to build a monument to something greater and more lasting than the mere span of it? Are you seizing the opportunities of today? Are you doing all that you can to make your life count? Or could you do more?

Life is a question. What will your answer be?

14

Why is There Evil in the World?

They were two empty human husks, without souls, without mercy, killing for killing's sake.

Arriving at Columbine High School in Littleton, Colorado, at about 11:30 A.M., the two armed teenagers seemed no different from their classmates who were either eating lunch or going to fifth-period classes. No one had any reason to think that April 20, 1999, would be anything but another ordinary day at school. But before the two killers had finished their bloody work and turned their guns upon themselves, twelve students and one teacher would be dead. Others would be wounded, even paralyzed for life.

Why is there such evil in the world? How can God—if there is a God—allow such a thing to happen?

The hard questions of Columbine

It was just five months later that my teenage daughter and I stood in a room with over three thousand other people to hear Darrell Scott recall that awful day. His daughter Rachel was the first to die. His son Craig was in the school library while ten of his classmates were executed around him. Craig survived by lying motionless in the blood of his best friend.

Darrell Scott described going into Columbine High School for the first time after the killings. "It was a war zone," he said. "I walked into that library and saw things that should never be seen in a high school. I was there before they had removed the blood. I wanted to experience just a little of what my son had to go through."

There was a painful ache in my own chest as I listened to this father recall the sweet, kind spirit of his slain daughter in a series of touching vignettes. He told about a Columbine student who was born with a physical deformity. The other kids had cruelly nicknamed him "Alien" because of his appearance and speech impediment. Several weeks after the killings, this boy went to Darrell Scott and, with tears in his eyes, told him, "Rachel was always nice to me. Every day, she put her arm around me and said, 'How are you doing today?'"

The morning of the tragedy, just an hour before she was killed, Rachel had put her arm around this boy, called him by name, and said, "I'm going to take you to a movie someday. We're going to get some coffee and have a good time." The boy concluded, "Every night since she died, I cry and I cry, because Rachel was the only person in school who was nice to me."

During his talk, Darrell Scott gave a PowerPoint presentation, flashing photos of the Columbine martyrs on a screen. First was Rachel Scott, seventeen. "My precious daughter," he said, "was one of two people killed outside the school building. They shot her as she was sitting just outside of the school, eating lunch. They shot her in the leg and she stood up to run, so they shot her through the chest. Then they turned their guns on Richard Castaldo, a young man right beside Rachel, and they shot him eight or nine times. He's paralyzed, and he attends Columbine today in a wheelchair.

"They went down some stairs to the cafeteria where they had planted several bombs. There were two big butane tanks with timers set to explode. The timers had failed to go off, so they shot at the tanks. Still they didn't explode. If they had, there would've been over four hundred fifty people killed.

"The boys came back outside and one of them went to my daughter, who was lying on the ground. He lifted her head up by her hair and said, 'Do you still believe in God?' She had talked to both boys about God three weeks before the rampage. She answered, 'Yes, I do.' And the last words she heard were, 'Then go be with Him.' And they shot her through the temple."

Danny Rohrbough, fifteen, was also killed outside the building. "Danny was a brave young man," said Scott, "who laid down his life for his friends. He had already escaped, but he turned and went back to the cafeteria. He was killed as he held the exit door open."

William "Dave" Sanders, forty-seven, was a business and computer teacher. When the shooting began, he shielded escaping students with his body. Shot twice in the chest, he bled to death over a three-hour period. "As he lay dying," said Scott, "students took the photos from his wallet and held them up before his eyes. He went into eternity looking at the pictures of his wife and two daughters."

The rest—ten in all—were killed in the library. As Craig described the scene to his father, the fifty kids in the library were startled by the sound of something splatting against the library door. Craig was sitting with his friend Matt at a table. Hearing the noise, they assumed it was a prank. But when a student stumbled in and fell onto the floor, bleeding from a gunshot wound, the kids dove under their desks. Matt and Craig huddled under one desk. Another boy, Isaiah Shoels, was running, looking for a place to hide, but all the desks were taken. Craig yelled, "Isaiah, get down here with us!" So Matt, Craig, and Isaiah crowded together under the desk.

Seconds later, the gunmen entered the library. Their first victim: Kyle Velasquez, sixteen, a six-foot-tall "gentle giant," as Darrell Scott called him. He had been insecure most of his life because of a learning disability. Normally, he wouldn't have been on campus at that time, but he had recently started going to the library on his lunch break to use the computers. About six months before he died, Kyle's parents noticed that this once-insecure boy had come to a place of contentment with himself and his life.

After shooting Kyle, the killers began asking kids in the library if they believed in God. One girl, Valerie Schnurr, eighteen, said, "Yes, I do." The gunmen shot her nine times. Amazingly, she survived. The killers asked another girl, Kacey Ruegsegger, seventeen, if she believed in God. She, too, answered yes—then hid her face and waited to die. "I could feel the evil in that room," Kacey later recalled. "Yet, under my computer table, I could feel God or an angel with me." They shot Kacey multiple times, and she survived wounds in the shoulder, hands, throat, and face.[1]

The gunmen crouched low and sprayed bullets under the library desks. One of those killed was John Tomlin, sixteen. The previous summer, John had gone to Mexico with a church group, building houses for the poor. He died shielding another student with his body. Also killed was Steven Curnow, fourteen, a freshman who dreamed of piloting an

F-16 as a Navy top gun. He could recite every line from all the *Star Wars* movies.

Also killed: Kelly Fleming, sixteen, an aspiring poet and songwriter. Though she had always been shy, six months previously she had gone to her father and said, "Dad, I'm not going to be shy anymore." From then on, she was a changed person. Also killed: Lauren Townsend, eighteen, a senior and captain of the girls' varsity volleyball team. Lauren would have been the valedictorian at her graduation. Her mother accepted her diploma instead.

Also killed: Daniel Mauser, fifteen, a straight-A student who excelled in math, science, and cross-country. He had recently spent two weeks in Paris with his French club. Also killed: Corey DePooter, seventeen, a kid who loved to golf, hunt, and fly-fish. "Corey's grave is next to my daughter's," said Darrell Scott. "He was shot several times and couldn't have an open casket, so he was cremated. I see his grave often, and all of his friends come to the grave and leave fly-fishing equipment, vests, and rod-and-reels."

The killers walked across the room and selected their next victim: Cassie Bernall, seventeen. Once a nihilistic teenager without a goal in life, she had recently become a born-again Christian and turned her life around. She fell dead about ten feet from where Craig, Matt, and Isaiah huddled together.

The killers spotted Isaiah Shoels, eighteen. Though physically small (four feet, ten inches, 120 pounds), Isaiah was a good football player and a weight-lifter who could bench-press twice his own weight. He was the only African American to die in the rampage. "There's that little n——— son of a bitch right there!" the killers shouted. "Let's get him!" They cursed Isaiah with every obscenity and racial slur they could think of. Those were the last words Isaiah heard before they shot him in the head, execution-style.

Then the killers turned their guns on Matthew Kechter, sixteen. Matt was a defensive tackle on the JV squad. The killers targeted him because he wore a baseball cap and a football jersey. "Get any f——ing jock!" the killers said.

Craig was sure he was next. He put his head down in the spreading blood of his friends and waited to die. "I was scared," Craig later told his father. "I just knew they were standing over me. Finally, I prayed and said, 'God, take away my fear.' And instantly, I wasn't afraid. I knew right then that God was real, because my prayer was answered. And I heard God speak inside me as clearly as if He were in that room: 'Get up and get out!'" Craig lifted his head, expecting to see the killers—but there was no one around him but the dead and wounded.

Craig called, "Let's get out of here!" He went to Kacey Ruegsegger and lifted her to her feet—most of her shoulder was blown away—and he put her good arm around his neck and led the survivors out of the school building and into the parking lot. Without realizing it, he passed within a few feet of the body of his sister Rachel.

After memorializing each Columbine martyr, Darrell Scott posed a question to the audience: "How many of you believe there is a God?" Every hand in the auditorium went up. "How many of you believe that God is in control?" The upraised hands wavered uncertainly.

"I believe God is in control," Darrell Scott said. "I believe God is almighty and all-powerful. I believe He knows the end from the beginning. But I'll tell you something: Those questions are a lot harder to answer when your daughter is dead."

Putting God on trial

We don't have to go back to the Holocaust to find soul-shattering, mind-numbing evil. It was there in the upscale Denver suburb of Littleton, Colorado.

Evil was also stalking Huff Creek Road outside of Jasper, Texas, where three white men beat a black man, James Byrd, Jr., then chained him to the rear bumper of a pickup truck. They dragged him for two miles at high speeds until his head and one arm were ripped from his body.

Evil was in Wyoming when Matthew Shepard, a twenty-one-year-old college student, was kidnapped, robbed, pistol-whipped until his skull caved in, tortured with cigarettes, and taunted as he begged for his life. It took him a long time to die, alone and suffering, tied to a fence in near-freezing temperatures. He was hated and killed because he was different.

Evil overshadowed one of the most beautiful places in the world, Yosemite National Park, when a thrill-killer kidnapped, tortured, and murdered female sightseers Carole and Juli Sund and foreign exchange student Silvina Pelosso; he also killed and beheaded a Yosemite naturalist, Joie Ruth Armstrong.

Of course, the evil that we human beings inflict on one another is not the only kind of evil in the universe. When we ask ourselves how a good and powerful God could allow evil in the world, we must also address such issues as pain and injustice. How could a loving God allow a little child to suffer and die from leukemia? Why would a good and just God allow evil people to prosper while good people struggle to exist? Such questions have converted many to agnosticism and atheism.

In 1940, C. S. Lewis published *The Problem of Pain*, a series of logical and well-reasoned rationales explaining how a loving God could create a world filled with evil and pain. But twenty years after that book was published, Lewis lost his wife Joy to cancer. It had been a long and agonizing illness, and her suffering had caused him to question many of the tidy religious certainties of *The Problem of Pain*.

Lewis journaled his feelings of loss, and his journal was published in 1961 as *A Grief Observed*. The book was so angry in its questioning of God that Lewis originally had it published under the pseudonym "N. W. Clerk" (a pun on the Old English for "I know not what scholar"). Though *A Grief Observed* ultimately takes the reader to a place of reassurance, it begins with the most disturbing of doubts:

> Not that I am (I think) in much danger of ceasing to believe in God. The real danger is of coming to believe such dreadful things about Him. The conclusion I dread is not, "So there's no God after all," but, "So this is what God's really like. Deceive yourself no longer."[2]

We skim the surface of life, thinking of our pleasure and amusement, the status and possessions we want, the career goals we pursue. Then some horror comes crashing into our lives—an illness, the death of a close friend or family member, a devastating accident. Suddenly, we are forced to look deeper into our souls. We ask why God hides from us when our need is greatest? Is God uncaring? Is God cruel? Is God nonexistent?

The attempt to reconcile the existence of a good God with the reality of evil is called *theodicy*. In a world where God is on trial for the crime of permitting evil in the world, theodicy is counsel for the defense. But the prosecutor seems to have all the evidence on his side. The logic of the case seems irrefutable: If God is all-powerful and there is evil in the world, then God must be evil. But if God is all-good and there is evil in the world, then God must be impotent. As Archibald MacLeish observed in his 1958 play *J.B.*, based on the biblical story of Job: "If God is God, He is not good; if God is good, He is not God."

When a child dies of leukemia, what is our response? Some say, "The child will go to Heaven." Okay—but does this justify the child's pain and death? Is it right and good for God to allow such suffering, Heaven or no Heaven? It hardly seems so. Some say, "It's all part of God's plan." Really? What good and merciful plan would allow such suffering and evil? Certainly an all-wise God could devise a better plan than that. Some say, "God never gives us more than we can handle." But from what I've seen, the world is filled with suffering that is intolerable by any rational definition.

Some say, "We need bad things in the world as a contrast, so we will appreciate the good." But if I am admiring a beautiful sunset, I do not think, "Isn't this a wonderful contrast to war and cancer and AIDS!" I simply enjoy the beauty and goodness of the sunset for its own sake. Some say, "Suffering is a punishment for sin." Then why do so many good people suffer? Some say that human beings stand guilty before God. Others say that God stands guilty before humanity.

Is God in control? Despite the death of his daughter and the terrifying ordeal of his son, Darrell Scott says yes, God is in control. But what does God control? Certainly God does not control human choices, such as the choices of the Columbine killers. If God is in control, then that control is exercised very broadly and loosely.

So how does God exercise control of a world in which human free will reigns? At best, God rules over a rebellious kingdom—and God does not seem to rein in the rebels among us. Evil people run riot. They kill and maim and torture, and no bolt of lightning, not even a voice from heaven, intervenes.

If God is the author of everything, then mustn't God be the author of evil, too? If God has the whole world in his hands, then aren't the hands of God stained with the blood of millions? Edmund Burke once said, "The only thing necessary for evil to triumph is for good men to do nothing." Very true—but if evil triumphs when good *men* do nothing, how much more must evil triumph when a good *God* does nothing? That is why the French essayist Stendhal remarks, "The only excuse for God is that He does not exist."

Atheists will tell you with absolute certainty that the existence of evil proves the impossibility of God. The argument goes like this:

1. If God exists, then meaningless pain and evil cannot exist; a good and powerful God would not allow it.
2. We know that meaningless pain and evil *do* exist.
3. Therefore, God does *not* exist.

Sounds logical. But the problem with that little formulation is that we, being limited human beings, cannot possibly know with certainty whether God (if there is a God) has logical, moral reasons for allowing bad things to happen to good people. Suffering that seems meaningless and pointless to us might have meaning and a valid justification in the eternal scheme of things. "Is it not conceivable," asks Auschwitz survivor Viktor Frankl, "that there is still another dimension, a world beyond man's world; a world in which the question of an ultimate meaning of human suffering would find an answer?"[3] Frankl has the authority to ask such a question. But even if the answer is yes, it is cold comfort if the suffering we are talking about is, say, the death of a child.

Free will: "the ultimate human reality"

Near the end of the 1981 movie *Time Bandits*, there is a scene of enormous carnage and mayhem inflicted on the world by the satanic Evil Genius (David Warner). After all the dust settles and the Evil Genius is vanquished by the Supreme Being (Sir Ralph Richardson), it is time to take stock and figure out the moral to the movie. So the young boy in the film, Kevin (Craig Warnock), questions the Supreme Being about all the death and destruction that has just taken place. "You mean," says Kevin, "you let all those people die—just to test your creation?"

"Yes, you really are a clever boy," replies the Supreme Being.

"Why did they have to die?" asks Kevin.

The Supreme Being shrugs. "You might as well say, 'Why do we have to have evil?'"

"Yes," says Kevin, "why do we have to have evil?"

"Ah!" says the Supreme Being. "I think it has something to do with free will."[4]

Free will! Yes, that's the heart of the issue of evil. Perhaps we can't ascribe *all* the pain and suffering in the world to human free will. For example, we can't say that a devastating earthquake or a case of childhood leukemia is somehow caused by human choice. But most of what we call "evil" in the world today is the *direct* result of human choices. It's a simple matter of cause and effect.

Of course, there are some who do not consider human free will a valid defense for God. Writing in *The American Atheist*, Martin L. Bard says that "if there is a god, he is intensely cruel." Bard cites the tribal wars in Rwanda in the spring of 1994. More than five hundred thousand people—including at least one hundred thousand children—were butchered, most of them hacked to death. Bard reflects:

> This was one of many sickening genocidal events in the terrible history of the world. God did nothing. He who supposedly had the power to prevent all of the suffering hindered none of it....By what great irrationality can we possibly believe that there is a god who, having completely neglected those precious, mutilated children, nevertheless has concern for us? …
>
> If we had ultimate power we would not permit any suffering. How can it be that a god is less kind than we?[5]

This, of course, is not a new question. But the logic of the matter is really quite clear: As human beings, we cannot have free will without the possibility of evil. Those who would have God create a world in which we have free will but no potential for evil might as well demand that God create a round square. Either human beings *must* be nothing more than programmed robots, or there *must* be the potential for humans to do evil things. There is no third alternative.

In *People of the Lie*, psychiatrist M. Scott Peck says, "Free will is the ultimate human reality....Evil is the inevitable concomitant of free will, the price we pay for our unique human power of choice."[6] But what a price! Rivers of blood, the cries of butchered children! Surely, God should revoke our terrible freedom and stop the suffering and madness of the human condition. Yet, in the cosmic scheme of things, there appears to be some reason beyond our understanding why God refuses to violate human freedom. God (if there is a God) will not force us to be good, even to prevent a holocaust. Peck concludes:

Having forsaken force, God is impotent to prevent the atrocities that we commit upon one another. He can only continue to grieve with us. He will offer us Himself in all His wisdom, but He cannot make us choose to abide with Him.

For the moment, then, God, tormented, waits upon us through one holocaust after another.[7]

Who, then, is responsible for the suffering that is caused by human free will? Is it God? Or is it—us?

There is an old parable that underscores our own responsibility for the evil in the world. In this story, a man goes to God in prayer and complains about all the suffering and injustice in the world. "God," he says, "why do you allow this to go on? Why don't you send help?"

"I did send help," God replies. "I sent you."

What about natural evil?

Although the human mind recoils from the horrors of the Holocaust or Rwanda or Columbine, we recognize that these tragedies are the direct result of human free will. God didn't stoke the fires of Auschwitz or butcher the victims of Rwanda or go on a rampage at Columbine. Human beings did.

But what about *natural evil*—the evil in the world that has nothing to do with human free will? If a lifelong smoker contracts lung cancer, we can see a clear element of human choice in that illness—but the eight-year-old child with leukemia did nothing to bring on her disease. Isn't God directly responsible for that child's suffering?

And what about killer earthquakes and other so-called "acts of God"? These cataclysmic forces of nature clearly have no connection with human free will. It could be argued that human beings make the choice whether or not to live in earthquake-prone areas. For example, in 1994, the 6.7-magnitude Northridge quake killed seventy-two people in the Los Angeles area and caused $40 billion in damage; in 1999, however, a more powerful 7.1-magnitude quake rocked southern California but killed no one and caused comparatively little damage. Why? Because the more powerful quake was centered near Joshua Tree, in a sparsely populated desert.

You might say that if people choose to live in earthquake-prone regions, they accept a certain risk. Yet there are risks of natural disasters wherever you choose to live—risks of tornadoes, floods, hurricanes, blizzards, heat waves, sink holes, and more. Choosing to live where disaster might strike is not an immoral or evil choice.

So we are back to the question of how a good and loving God could create a world with natural evil. Take, for example, the Izmit, Turkey, quake in August 1999. That 7.4 quake killed seventeen thousand people, and was the worst in Turkey since a December 1939 quake that killed thirty-three thousand. Many of the buildings

> "*As human beings, we cannot have free will without the possibility of evil.*"

that collapsed in the Izmit quake were built in recent years to modern earthquake-resistant standards (Turkish building codes are very similar to safety codes in California). But many of the buildings in and around Izmit were laterally shifted *ten feet* in a single, sudden jolt. Few buildings, no matter how well engineered, could withstand such a shock.

Why do earthquakes happen? Because of a natural geological process called *plate tectonics*. Believe it or not, the process of plate tectonics has a lot to do with understanding the problem of natural evil. Bear with me. I think you'll find this interesting.

The word *tectonics* comes from the Greek word *tekton*, meaning "builder." Plate tectonics is the study of how the earth's crust is built of a series of interlocking plates. These plates are under stress due to heat and movement deep within the Earth. The Earth's core, composed mostly of iron, is thought to be about twelve thousand degrees Fahrenheit, due to radioactivity within the planet. Wrapped around that hot core is the Earth's mantle, composed of viscous rock—the same molten rock that is emitted from volcanoes in the form of lava.

The immense heat within the earth causes convection currents of molten rock in the mantle. Over long periods of time, these currents slowly rise, rupture the crust, and carry plates of the crust along. The tectonic plates grind against each other, snag on each other, and sometimes break loose with devastating force—an earthquake. Sometimes, the break in the crust allows molten rock from the mantle to vent and spew above ground—a volcano. What we think of as "solid" terra firma is really nothing more than a thin skin of floating rock. Just a few miles below our feet is a hellish underworld of molten, radioactive slag in a constant state of slow boil.

The land mass of Turkey is unfortunately located at the junction of several major tectonic plates—the African, Arabian, Iranian, and Eurasian plates. Izmit is on the western extension of the North Anatolian fault, an active region at the edge of the Eurasian tectonic plate. So if you are looking for a reason the Izmit quake killed seventeen thousand people in the summer of 1999, the reason is simple: plate tectonics.

A person who believes in God might well ask, "Why did God create such a cruel world of plate tectonics, earthquakes, and volcanoes? Why didn't God place us in a world without seismic activity? I would much rather live in a world where earthquakes can never happen."

No, you wouldn't. In fact, you couldn't. The same process of plate tectonics that produces killer quakes and killer volcanoes also makes life possible on Planet Earth. Without plate tectonics, our planet would be a dead world. What seems evil at first glance is actually necessary for life to exist.

In their book *Rare Earth*, geologist Peter D. Ward and astronomer Donald Brownlee explain several life-giving functions of plate tectonics. The most important one is this:

Plate tectonics gives rise to volcanoes, and volcanoes vent carbon dioxide (CO_2), a "greenhouse gas." Greenhouse gases are gases composed of three or more atoms (other greenhouse gases include water vapor, ozone, and methane). These gases trap infrared energy to warm the planet. If it weren't for greenhouse gases, the oceans would freeze and life on Earth would end.

Tectonic plates and the volcanoes they cause are part of a complex process that acts as a "global thermostat." It's a fascinating cycle. Volcanoes emit CO_2. On the surface of the planet, the CO_2 chemically combines with calcium silicate found in common weathered rocks (such as granite), forming calcium carbonate (the primary constituent of limestone) and silicon dioxide. Rain and weathering wash the calcium carbonate into the ocean, where (by a process called "subduction") it is absorbed down into the Earth's crust. There, the carbonates decompose, releasing CO_2, which is eventually vented out through volcanoes again.

This cycle is amazingly well regulated and sensitive to changes in atmospheric temperature. When the Earth warms, the rate of chemical weathering increases, causing more CO_2 to be removed from the atmosphere. Result: The Earth cools. As the planet cools, weathering decreases, causing more CO_2 to be retained in the atmosphere. Result: The Earth warms up. In this cyclical fashion, the Earth oscillates between warm and cool, just like a thermostat turning the furnace of a house on and off in response to changing temperatures. The entire cycle depends on plate tectonics to keep the volcanoes spewing their CO_2 and to keep minerals exposed so the weathering process can occur. If plate tectonics ceased, the thermostatic cycle would shut down, the planet would freeze, and life would end.

The price we pay for living on this beautiful planet is an occasional earthquake. To those who suffer in such disasters, plate tectonics must seem like an evil thing. But in the bigger picture, the process of plate tectonics is a good thing, a life-giving thing. If plate tectonics is a natural evil, it is also a *necessary* evil, because we can't live without it.

Let's look at another example of natural evil. We think of pain itself as an evil thing. Wouldn't life be better if there were no pain in the world? Yet there are people who do not experience pain—and you would not envy them. They are people with leprosy.

There is a common misconception that leprosy has been eradicated from the world. Fact is, according to the World Health Organization, there are over four million people with leprosy in the world today—most of them in India. Fortunately, the disease is now curable with modern anti-biotics.

Until recently, leprosy was thought of as a disease that directly caused lesions, blindness, and the loss of fingers, toes, hands, and feet. But thanks to the pioneering research of Dr. Paul Brand, an English physician who grew up in India, we now understand that leprosy is a bacterial infection that attacks the nerves under the skin, causing a loss of the ability to feel pain.

Because a person afflicted with leprosy feels no pain, injuries go unnoticed and untreated. If a person with leprosy gets a skin laceration, he is not aware when it becomes infected. If he sprains an ankle, he feels nothing and keeps walking on it. He has no sensation of dryness in the eyes, so he doesn't blink, and his unlubricated corneas become damaged by grit. Fingers and toes are not lost to degeneration but to wounds, burns, and infections that fester without attention. Why? Because leprosy sufferers have lost the protective benefit of what Dr. Brand calls "the gift of pain."

Pain is not the mindless blunder of blind evolution or an uncaring Creator. Properly understood, pain is a bioengineering marvel. It's as essential to our well-being as our five senses, our circulatory system, or our immune system. Pain is an ingenious warning system that keeps us from burning our hand on the stove. The benefit of pain derives from the very fact that it is so unpleasant.

Of course, not all pain is beneficial. Usually, we can alleviate pain by treating the wound or disorder that caused the pain—but not always. The pain of terminal cancer, the pain of crippling arthritis, the pain of a migraine headache—these are examples of pain run amok. Despite advances in the science of pain management, there are times when it is difficult or impossible to "switch off" a person's pain. This kind of pain is tragic and senseless—but it doesn't negate the fact that *most* of the pain we experience serves a beneficial function.

We hate and fear pain. We consider pain one of the most evil experiences imaginable. Yet pain is a vital mechanism, ensuring our health and survival. The example of leprosy teaches us that a pain-free life is a crippled life.

Consider another example of natural evil. Our planet coalesced into existence some four and a half billion years ago. Life arose not long afterward, evolving and diversifying over the next few billions of years. For about 150 million years, dinosaurs ruled the planet. Then, about sixty-five million years ago, a massive comet struck the Earth at a place we now know as the Yucatan in Mexico. The impact blasted a crater some one hundred twenty-five miles in diameter and exterminated 85 percent of life on the planet. The most dramatic result was that every single dinosaur species was wiped out.

From the dinosaurs' point of view, this event was a genocidal evil. But from our point of view, it was a good thing. The mass extinction of the dinosaurs enabled the emergence of the mammals—including, eventually, the human species. Was the comet strike in the Yucatan a random accident—or an act of God? Did God *deliberately* wipe out the dinosaurs to enable the emergence of intelligent human life? If so, was God good to do so? Or was it an evil thing to render the dinosaurs extinct? Sometimes in the natural world it is difficult to know good from evil.

Most people would consider a forest fire an evil thing. Yet, to the giant sequoia tree, a forest fire is the breath of life.

I recently visited the Mariposa Grove of giant sequoias near Yosemite National Park and stood in the presence of some of the oldest living things on Earth. There is a cathedral-like silence throughout that old-growth forest, and to stand in that grove is a spiritual experience. The eldest of all the giant sequoias (over 2,700 years old) is the Grizzly Giant, which was an ancient standing timber when Christ was born. Nearly 210 feet tall and over 30 feet in diameter, with a massive burn scar at its base, the Grizzly Giant has survived lightning storms, droughts, and uncounted forest fires. Yet it is still alive, its boughs still green. It's the most majestic tree I've ever seen, yet there is also

> "God didn't stoke the fires of Auschwitz or butcher the victims of Rwanda or go on a rampage at Columbine. Human beings did."

an air of fragility about it. Though its root system spreads out over more than three acres, the roots are close to the surface and easily damaged.

Fire is the key to the survival of these trees. During most of the twentieth century, we "protected" these trees from forest fires, not realizing we were killing them with kindness. With all fires carefully suppressed by the U.S. Forestry Service, the sequoias could not reproduce. Hardly any seedlings took root during the entire first half of the twentieth century. Entire cycles of sequoia reproduction came and went, and no new seedlings sprouted.

Then in 1977, a managed burn in the Kings Canyon National Park got out of control, scorching a two-acre section of sequoia groves. Many ancient trees were blackened and scarred—but not destroyed. In fact, the trees actually experienced a growth spurt after the fire. Sequoia seedlings soon sprouted. Conservationists learned that fire was the sequoias' natural friend, for it burned off competing shrubs and trees, and opened the sequoia cones so that the seeds would fall. The species actually *depended* on forest fires to survive. To deprive the ancient trees of fire was to do them great harm.

So what seems "evil" from a limited human perspective is often actually good from a deeper, broader perspective.

But what about the natural evil of catastrophic disease? Is God to blame when a little child is stricken with leukemia? Is God to blame when the personality of a beloved grandfather slowly disintegrates due to the ravages of Alzheimer's disease? I have no rational, logical answers for this kind of natural evil. But there may be an answer nonetheless. In *Denial of the Soul*, M. Scott Peck suggests just such an answer:

I defy you in your imagination to concoct a more ideal environment for human learning than this life on earth. It is a life filled with vicissitudes and existential suffering, but as Benjamin Franklin said, "Those things that hurt, instruct." Many have referred to earth as a vale of tears. Keats, however, went deeper when he called it "The vale of soul-making...."

No work I ever did as a psychotherapist was as fulfilling to me as that with a number of dying patients. People tend to learn best when they have a deadline....Dying can be the opportunity of a lifetime for learning and soul development.[8]

If you do not believe in God, then you have no complaint against God for the pain, evil, and injustice of this world. An imaginary God is no more responsible for the state of the world than Santa Claus or the tooth fairy.

But if you do believe in God, then you probably believe in the proposition that there is more to our existence than this brief span of years. If you believe, then you know that this life, with its pain and baffling evils, can become a vale of soul-making. It all depends on the attitude with which we face life and death. This is a world in which God does not seem to restrain human free will or natural evil. Yet those who believe in the reality of God are convinced that evil does not have the last word.

Rachel's diary

My daughter and I stood at the back of the balcony as Darrell Scott talked about the death of his daughter Rachel. There were over three thousand people in that auditorium, filling not only the seats but the aisles, the doorways, and the lobby. There were tears on the faces of the people around me. I vividly recall the chill I felt in my spine—that sensation you feel in the presence of something awesome and mysterious. I experienced that sensation near the close of Darrell Scott's talk, as he told us the most amazing story—the story of Rachel's diary.

"Rachel died and left us with things that I knew had to be shared with people," he said. "For a year and half before the Columbine killings, God was preparing Rachel's heart, and she wrote about it in her diary." Rachel's diary was in her backpack at the time she was killed, so for weeks it remained in the possession of the sheriff's department. Rachel's grieving parents desperately wanted that diary, because it contained the last recorded thoughts and feelings of their daughter.

Several weeks after Rachel's funeral, Darrell Scott received a call from a wealthy businessman in Ohio. "I saw your daughter's funeral on CNN," the man said, "and I sense that God wants me to financially support you so that you can go around the country and talk to people about how God is changing lives through this tragedy."

Well, that surprised Darrell Scott. He had been experiencing a growing sense that God was going to somehow bring good out of this tragedy, but he didn't know how. The man from Ohio had just given him an inkling.

"But that's not the real reason I'm calling," the man continued. "The reason I wanted to talk to you is because I had a dream. Three times in my life I've had dreams I knew were from God. The first two had to do with my businesses; both times they came to pass. This third dream was about your daughter. I dreamed I saw tears coming from Rachel's eyes, and her tears were watering something—but I couldn't see what. So I had to call and ask if it means anything to you."

"No," said Darrell Scott. "No, it really doesn't mean anything to me." Scott later asked his family and several of Rachel's friends. No one knew what the man's dream meant.

Five days passed. The sheriff's department called. "We're ready to release your daughter's backpack," they said. So Darrell Scott drove to the sheriff's office, retrieved the backpack, and hurried back to his pickup. Sitting behind the steering wheel, he took out the one thing that mattered most: Rachel's bullet-scarred diary.

He flipped to the last page Rachel had written—and his stunned eyes filled with tears. "I was more shocked by what I saw there," he told the audience, "than by anything else that has ever happened to me, including her death. I couldn't move. I just sat there in my truck and wept for more than thirty minutes. I prayed, 'God! You've got to tell me what this means!'"

> "If you do not believe in God, then you have no complaint against God for the pain, evil, and injustice of this world. An imaginary God is no more responsible for the state of the world than Santa Claus or the tooth fairy."

But it wasn't until over a month after retrieving Rachel's diary that Darrell Scott learned the full meaning of his daughter's final diary entry. It was not written in words. It was a drawing. It turned out that Rachel's best friend, Sarah, was with Rachel when she made that drawing, no more than thirty minutes before she was killed. Sarah said that Rachel had been drawing rapidly, intensely, as if her life depended on finishing that picture.

It was a picture of Rachel's tears.

Darrell Scott put the picture on the PowerPoint display. A gasp went through the room. A tingle went through my soul.

Rachel had drawn her own eyes, and dropping from her eyes were thirteen tears—*just as there were thirteen martyrs of the Columbine tragedy*. The tears watered a rose, and the rose grew out of the middle of a flowering columbine plant. This was the picture that Rachel had been drawing so furiously, as if her life depended on it, just minutes before her death.

Darrell Scott found many other astounding entries in Rachel's diary. There were lines of deeply expressive poetry his daughter had written—lines that seemed to suggest that Rachel actually had a premonition that her life would be cut short. "I have a purpose, I have a dream," said one couplet. "I have a future—or so it seems." And another: "All I want is for someone to walk with me / Through these halls of a tragedy." And on May 2, 1998, just eleven and a half months before her death, she made an entry consisting of three short sentences: "This will be my last year, Lord. I have gotten what I can. Thank you."

Darrell Scott is convinced God gave his daughter a vision, and that she set down that vision in her diary. He is convinced that God gave a fragment of this same vision to a man in Ohio. "I asked God, 'What does this mean?'" said Darrell Scott, "and God has gently spoken to my spirit. I understand now. That rose symbolizes all the changed lives that God is raising up out of this Columbine tragedy. I believe God is raising young people up out of the ashes of this tragedy to do a great work for their generation."

Seeing how many lives have been so profoundly affected by the life and death of Rachel Scott—including my own—it is hard for me to argue with that conclusion. How could anyone make sense of something as senseless as the murder of children? Yet, in the case of Rachel Scott, good has arisen from the ashes of evil. And that is something to cling to.

When Rachel Scott left this world, she bequeathed a last will and testament, a hastily drawn image of thirteen tears falling to the ground, and a rose springing up out of the grief and sadness. That rose is our hope in a world of incomprehensible evil and tragedy.

This may not be a fully satisfying answer, but I believe it is a true answer. And it is the only answer we have.

15

How Can I Get Past My Fear of Death?

Some years ago, when I drove to the library or the grocery store, I would sometimes notice an old man pedaling a bicycle along the palm-lined avenue. He made quite a visual impression, with his heavy eyebrows and distinctive walrus mustache. I saw him several times, but it never occurred to me to stop my car, get out, and talk to him. It wasn't until some months after his death that I learned who that man was: William Saroyan, one of the greatest writers of the twentieth century.

I've often wondered how my life would have been impacted if I had tried to get to know this man—if I had just taken a few moments to stop and introduce myself, to ask him about the life of a writer, to gather a little sage advice from the author of *The Human Comedy* and *The Time of Your Life*. Maybe he would have said, "Get away, kid! Don't bother me!" (as another writer, Robert Heinlein, once told me—or words to that effect). At least that would have given me a story to tell. But to have completely bypassed the chance to meet him—what a tragedy!

Five days before his death in 1981, Saroyan phoned Associated Press and made his final statement to the world: "Everybody has got to die, but I have always believed an exception would be made in my case. Now what?"

I think we are all like Saroyan. Sure, we know on some superficial level that everybody has to die—but we can't quite believe that it really applies to *us*. But a time comes when the inevitable can no longer be denied, when we must face our own mortality and ask ourselves: "Now what?"

A patch of death

One of my earliest memories goes back to the year 1955, when I was two and a half years old. My parents lived in one half of a duplex, and my Grandma and Grandpa Denney lived in the other half. Living so close to my grandparents, I got used to seeing them every day. I used to sit on my Grandpa Denney's lap and watch TV with him. My grandmother would fix me oatmeal with butter and brown sugar. I remember these things, though I was very small.

But the memory that made the strongest impression on me was of a particular day in December 1955. I knocked on my grandma's front door (since I was so little, my mother was probably with me, though I don't specifically recall). My grandmother opened the door, and I asked, "Where's Grandpa?"

"He's not here, Jimmy," she said. "He went to Heaven."

"When will he come home?" I asked.

"Heaven is Grandpa's home now," she said.

I still recall how puzzled I felt. Where is Heaven? And why did Grandpa go there? And why doesn't he come back? It didn't make any sense.

That was my first encounter with the mystery of death.

A few years later, when I was six, I was visiting at my cousins' house. I had three cousins, all girls, who lived on the next block (at that time, we all lived in a sleepy little central California oil-town, Coalinga). We were sitting around the dining room table, playing Chinese checkers. The older girls (Mary was eight and Gayle was seven) were engaged in a *big-kid* discussion, and I—terribly anxious to be a big kid, too—entered into the discussion as best I could.

I don't know how it came up, but for some reason Mary and Gayle were talking about death. Well, I knew *all* about people dying. I had watched *lots* of Westerns. "I'm not gonna die," I declared.

"Sure you will," said Mary.

"Will not!" I countered in my best know-it-all style. "I'm *not* gonna die! I'm a kid and kids don't die—just grownups." After all, the only people who died on TV were grownups—and *bad* grownups at that.

"Everybody has to die," said Gayle. "Someday you'll be a grownup and you'll die, too."

I could see I was on the losing end of this argument. My cousins seemed to know something I didn't—and that made me mad. I'm not sure if I was more mad about having to die someday or about losing an argument with know-it-all girls—but I do remember that the part about having to die struck me as grossly unfair. Still does, in fact.

A few years have passed, and I've learned something important: My cousins were right—I *am* going to die. I've tried to find some way around it, but there's no escaping it. So far, I haven't received a fatal diagnosis. I don't know *when* my death is going to happen. I don't know *how* it's going to happen. I just know it's going to happen, just as my cousins predicted.

And I hate to be the one to break this to you, but you're going to die, too. I'm sure this isn't the first time this thought has ever occurred to you. In fact, you've probably thought about it a lot.

I think about death nearly every day. I'm not morbid or despondent about it, but the subject is frequently on my mind. I think about the fact that, even if I live to be a hundred, I won't get to accomplish more than a fraction of the things I want to accomplish. There just aren't enough hours in a day, and there aren't enough days in a lifetime, to write all the books I have ideas for. If I lived to be a thousand years old, I'd just be getting started. I'd also like to travel and see more of the world. I'd like to visit the Moon and Mars. I'd like to study painting, take guitar lessons, learn to fly a plane. That's just for starters—my wish list is long. Some of the things I want to do I may eventually get around to; most, by far, I won't. Life is just too short.

As a matter of fact, death keeps me up at night—not the *fear* of death, exactly, but the *urgency* that death imposes on life. Death is the ultimate incentive. I don't like to go to sleep at night, because there's always *one more thing* I can get done if I stay up a little longer. I like being awake because I like being alive. Sleep, as Ray Bradbury once observed, is a patch of death.

A good day to die

We've all heard people say, "Death is just a part of life." Personally, I have no use for saccharine sentiments. Death may be a part of life, but it's certainly not the best part. Fact is, it's the part of life that shuts down all the other parts. It's the period at the end of a sentence.

The idea of death embodies all our greatest terrors: What if I die old and helpless? What if I die abandoned and alone? What if I die in pain or paralysis? What if I never find meaning in life, and my death is just the end of a meaningless existence? What if I die unforgiven, with guilt on my soul? What if I'm forgotten when I die? These are questions that keep us wide awake at three in the morning.

Death is an evil. It's a disfiguring knife-slash across the face of human existence. Death is not a thing to be accepted with syrupy platitudes and polite euphemisms. It is an obscenity, a thing to make the soul seethe with rage, as Dylan Thomas said: "Do not go gentle into that good night / Rage, rage against the dying of the light."

Yet while death is certain, fear of death is not inevitable. Once you have settled the question of death in your own soul, you are ready to truly *live*.

A cemetery is an excellent place to think about living. A funeral is a fine place to take a good, long look down our own road. But, over the years, I've been to a number of funerals—some great funerals and some terrible ones—and, on the whole, I've concluded that we don't do a very good job of dealing with death. Even at funerals, when the reality of death is rubbed in our faces, we retreat into denial. Uncle Henry is laid out in a casket that costs as much as a new Buick. He's surrounded by a Rose Parade of flowers, coated with more makeup than Tammy Faye Bakker and Mimi Bobeck combined, looking for all the world like an exhibit in a wax museum. The mourners pass by, whispering euphemisms of denial: Uncle Henry has "passed on" or "gone home." Geez, can't we just say the man is *dead*?

Our cowardly denial of our mortality makes us weak and pathetic, heightens our fear, and renders us all the more helpless and unprepared when it comes time to deal with a loved one's mortality—or our own. We *must* face the truth about death.

Death is not a good thing, but truth is. If we are courageous and honest with ourselves, there is always good that can come out of bad things, even a thing like death.

As dark and evil as death appears, I've come to a surprising conclusion (surprising to me, anyway): There *is* something good to be said for death. For one thing, our mortality forces us to think about what is important. As Samuel Johnson once observed, "Depend upon it, sir, when a man knows he is to be hanged in a fortnight, it concentrates his mind wonderfully." The reality of death demands of us that we deal realistically with the business of living—the meaning of life, the quality and value of the life we live, our relationships with loved ones, and our relationship with the Power behind the universe.

We should live each day with a light heart but "grave" minds, always conscious of our mortality. By staying connected with our mortality, we stay connected with living. As Rabbi Ben Kamin notes in *The Path of the Soul*, "A breath of death yields a good swallow of life."[1]

When we die, we have the opportunity to set an example for the next generation on how to live and how to die. One of my greatest fears about death—the thing I fear even more than the pain of the dying process—is the possibility that I might fail the test of dying well. I want to learn the lessons of living and dying, and I want to pass those lessons on to those who need my strength. If I have to die, I don't want to waste the opportunity to make something good of a bad thing.

> "Yet while death is certain, fear of death is not inevitable. Once you have settled the question of death in your own soul, you are ready to truly live."

So how does one do that? How do you prepare yourself to die well? The answer: *Live well*. By that I mean to live a life of courage, love, generosity, and good humor. Rabbi Kamin observes that the way people die usually reflects the way they have lived. In fact, death tends to intensify a person's traits: The person with a sweet personality usually dies sweetly; the angry, bitter person tends to die angrily and bitterly; the humorous person is funny to the end. "When somebody is dying," concludes Rabbi Kamin, "he or she is the same person, only more so."[2]

This is your life *right now*, and it is the proving ground for your death. So live *now*. Love those around you *now*. Build relationships that go deep, that can't be uprooted by time, change, and misfortune. Learn to trust; earn the trust of others. Invite a few close friends into the depths of your soul, and go deep into their souls, so that you are never truly alone. Prepare for your death by fully living your life. Savor past memories, look ahead to future joys—but above all, live fully in *today*, feasting on each fleeting moment, inhaling its sweetness.

Also, live each day with a continuous awareness of your connection to every other soul on the planet. Dr. Martin Luther King, Jr., once observed that we human beings are all "tied in a single garment of destiny. Whatever affects one directly affects all indirectly. I can never be what I ought to be until you are what you ought to be, and you can never be what you ought to be until I am what I ought to be." So live to serve others. Determine in your heart to leave this world in a little better shape than you found it.

If you live well *now*, then any day is a good day to die.

How to be Immortal

Should we resign ourselves to death—or is immortality possible? It all depends on what "immortality" means to you. Some years ago, novelist Michael P. Kube-McDowell posted the following observation on a CompuServe public forum:

> I have serious doubts that there's anything more to my personality and "selfness" than a synergy between genetics, neurochemistry, and the environments and experiences to which I've been exposed. And my expectation concerning death is that it will be both corporeal- and ego-death—which is part of the reason I write, to be honest. Like everyone who finds existence interesting and occasionally enjoyable, I want to live forever. And I'm pretty sure that "I" won't. The best I can do is to see that my genes live on through my children, and that my thoughts live on through my writing.[3]

To Kube-McDowell, the nearest thing to immortality he can imagine consists of creation and procreation—that is, writing and having children. Personally, I can empathize with him—but I can't agree with him. I love my children and I wouldn't trade being a father for anything in the world. But from the time they were born, they have been living their own individual lives. I hope I have helped to shape their values and their character, and I have tried to give them a good start in life. But to my mind, there is no meaningful sense in which I will "live on" through my children.

Can books make you immortal? Well, it's true that you can extend the shelf-life of your thoughts for decades, or even centuries, through books. Today, we can read the twenty-seven hundred-year-old thoughts of Homer and the four hundred-year-old thoughts of Shakespeare—but what are a few centuries next to genuine *immortality*? Fact is, paper deteriorates, bindings rot—there are few things more fragile in the world than books. Achieve immortality by writing books? No, I write because I feel I have something to say, and I want to get it said before I die, that's all. But books don't bestow immortality.

Before this day is over, a nuclear war or an asteroid from space could wipe away every recorded thought of Homer and Shakespeare, not to mention Michael P. Kube-McDowell and Jim Denney. In a few billion years, our Sun will expand, engulfing and destroying our Earth. Even if the human race escapes to a new and younger world, the universe itself will eventually die. Where will our genes and our thoughts be then?

I have no illusions about becoming immortal through my children or my books. Immortality, to me, does not consist of "making my mark on the world." Achievements and fame, my name in the history books, buildings named after me—what kind of immortality is that? The only kind of immortality that interests me is the kind where I don't have to die. Anything less, anything else, is not immortality at all.

Real Immortality—can we live forever?

Why must we die? "Well, that's obvious," you might say. "Nothing lives forever. All living things eventually succumb to old age."

But that's not true. Organisms that reproduce asexually (such as bacteria) do not die of old age. They reproduce by dividing, and they never age, never wear out, and never die unless they come in contact with a hostile environment (like a spritz of Lysol). The only organisms that die of old age are sexually reproducing organisms like ourselves. (And no, becoming celibate won't make you live longer. It'll just make life *seem* longer.)

Frank R. Zindler, science writer and former professor of biology at the State University of New York, observes that animal bodies—including our own human bodies—become disposable (from an evolutionary point of view) once reproductive activity is at an end. He writes:

> From a cost-benefit ratio point of view, maintaining animal bodies after the genes they carry have been passed on is wasteful. Just as a chicken is an egg's way of making another egg, an animal body is a device used by genes to insure successful reproduction and transmission through time. From this perspective, bodies are simply packaging for genes—wrappings to be discarded once the genes have "done their thing."[4]

So it would seem that death is the certain fate of all members of our species. But wait—Zindler goes on to cite recent research that suggests the possibility that scientists may soon learn how to "switch off" the body's aging/dying triggers (such as cellular oxidation), potentially halting and even reversing the aging and dying process.

The question naturally arises: Is that a good thing? "Well, of course it is!" you might say. "What could be wrong with ending death?" Consider this: Zindler suggests that immortality will likely be scientifically feasible within twenty years. That means that within our lifetime, we could be living in a world where nobody dies of old age. Presumably, however, people would continue to copulate—and copulation increases population. What if the older generation decides it will no longer make room for the next generation? What if the new immortals stubbornly elect to continue consuming precious space and resources? Does anyone else notice a potential problem here?

If, as Zindler suggests, biological immortality may be within our reach in a mere two decades or so, will the result be Heaven on Earth? Or a Hell of unbelievable overpopulation? Or will it be a brave new world in which immortality is rationed among the privileged few?

Against such a backdrop, does the death of an individual—even your death or mine—seem too high a price to pay to make room for our children and our children's children? Given this scenario, it's a price I would be willing to pay— albeit a bit begrudgingly. This is especially true in view of the evidence for the existence of God, the immortal soul, and the afterlife (as we will explore later). Frank R. Zindler scoffs at belief in an afterlife, which he sees as a pale substitute for physical immortality. He writes:

> Our religions, for the most part, have given up hope for physical immortality altogether and have invented "spiritual" immortality as a rather anemic substitute for which to hope....For millennia our superstitions have sold us an ersatz immortality and prevented us from seeking out the real one.[5]

But is "spiritual immortality" only an "ersatz" immortality as Zindler claims? Or could it be that physical immortality is merely an anemic substitute for the immortality we were *meant* to have? Which is the real immortality? Being physically alive in a dying, *Soylent Green* world? Or discovering, in the next moment after death, that the "ersatz immortality" Zindler disdains is in fact the *real* immortality we all secretly long for?

Let's be honest with ourselves: We all long for Heaven. Even those of us who don't believe in Heaven wish it were so. Frank Zindler writes glowingly about a future in which there is no more aging, no more death—and doesn't that sound like the Heaven of old?

All my life, I've been fascinated by two seemingly unrelated subjects—science fiction and spirituality. Recently, it occurred to me that these two areas of interest are not unrelated at all: The romance of space travel is just a symbolically disguised quest for God and Heaven. When atheists like Isaac Asimov, Carl Sagan, and Arthur C. Clarke write enthusiastically about the cosmos, and imagine radiant cities in space, vast civilizations among the stars, worlds without end, amen, *they are writing scientific descriptions of Heaven.*

When I treat my kids to a couple of days of carefree fun at Disneyland, or when we enjoy a perfect day at Yosemite or at the shores of the Pacific Ocean, I can't help thinking, *This is a little piece of Heaven.* Try to deny it. You know it's true. The longing for Heaven is inside of you, just as it's inside of me. In our intellectual pride, we have tried to banish all the "childish superstitions" and "religious myths" from our oh-so-educated minds—yet there is something inside us that seems to sense the absurdity of the notion that a human being is *here* one day and *gone* the next. On some level, we *know* that there is something about us that is truly immortal.

We die, yes—but we also live on. Some will deny it, and will go to their graves denying it. But I know it's true. Death is not the end. There is life after life. You don't have to believe it now. I've shown you no evidence—not yet—but I will do so by the end of this book. For the time being, I'll just say this: You and I have only one true hope for immortality. *Somehow, we must connect ourselves to the Infinite.* If our universe was designed by an infinite Creator, and if our souls are joined to that eternal Soul, how can we help but live forever?

"It's all a bunch of bull!"

With the publication of her 1969 book *On Death and Dying*, the Swiss-American physician Elisabeth Kübler-Ross made it possible for our society to openly discuss the once-undiscussible issues of the dying process. She was the first scientist to boldly investigate the end of life by actually sitting down with dying patients and asking them what they were going through. Out of her clinical observations came the now-famous Five Stages of Dying:

Stage 1: *Denial* ("Those can't be my lab tests! There must be some mistake!")

Stage 2: *Anger* ("God must be a monster to allow a thing like cancer to exist!" "What kind of lousy doctor are you that you didn't catch this sooner?")

Stage 3: *Bargaining* ("God, if You heal me, I'll quit drinking, be nice to my spouse, and go to church again!")

Stage 4: *Depression* ("My bargaining failed. I'm doomed. There is no hope.")

Stage 5: *Acceptance* ("Okay, I'm dying—but I refuse to waste the days I have left feeling bitter and sorry for myself.")

Obviously, people don't always progress through these stages in a neat, step-by-step sequence. Some go back and forth between stages. Some skip a stage. Some cycle through the stages multiple times. And some, quite tragically, get stuck in a stage like anger or depression—and that is where they die. Dr. Kübler-Ross did humanity an enormous favor in helping dying people and their caregivers understand the emotional process that occurs when a person learns he or she is about to die.

Dr. Kübler-Ross also led the fight to make care of the dying more humane, promoting hospice care and urging physicians to devote more attention to controlling pain and alleviating suffering. She pointed out the absurdity that physicians should withhold morphine from dying patients lest they become "drug addicts" in their final few days of life.

Over the years, Elisabeth Kübler-Ross sat at the bedside of literally thousands of dying people, including children, comforting them and listening to their stories and feelings. In the process, she came to believe in the immortality of the human soul and the goodness of a loving God who is there to ease our suffering and receive our souls at the end of life.

So it was a bitter irony that, in 1996, Dr. Kübler-Ross found herself crippled by a series of strokes, totally dependent on others—and stuck for months in the anger stage. In June 1997, partially paralyzed and anticipating her death, she vented her anger in an interview with reporter Don Lattin of the *San Francisco Chronicle*.

"For fifteen hours a day," she said, "I sit in this same chair, totally dependent on someone else coming in here to make me a cup of tea. It's neither living nor dying. It's stuck in the middle. My only regret is that for forty years I spoke of a good God who helps people, who knows what you need, and how all you have to do is ask for it. Well, that's baloney. I want to tell the world that it's a bunch of bull. Don't believe a word of it."

In the interview, Elisabeth Kübler-Ross described the deplorable conditions in which people were once forced to die. Arriving in America in 1958, she found that to die in an American hospital was a nightmare. Patients were not told they had cancer. They were put in a room at the end of the hall, ignored by the nurses, denied pain medication, and given no consolation for their fears and emotional needs. Over the years, care of the dying has greatly changed, to a large degree because of her efforts. But when Dr. Kübler-Ross herself was hospitalized, she wondered if anything had changed at all.

"It was like my work was nonexistent," she told Lattin. "The nurses never came to see their patients. They would just sit out there in front of their computers." Due to the strokes, she had paralysis and intense pain in one arm. "If you blew on my arm," she said, "I would scream." On one occasion, a fiendishly insensitive nurse remarked that Dr. Kübler-Ross was holding her hand in an odd way (which is common with stroke patients)—and the nurse proceeded to *sit* on her arm. "I slugged her with my good arm," Dr. Kübler-Ross recalled, "and I yelled, 'That hurts like hell!' She said, 'Oh, you're becoming combative,' and brought in two fat nurses who tried to sit on it again. If I'd had a pistol, I would have shot them."[6]

No wonder she was angry, bitter, and depressed in June 1997.

But two months later, Elisabeth Kübler-Ross gave another interview to a different reporter—and the tone of this interview contrasted starkly with the previous one. Talking to Cathy Hainer of *USA Today*, she said that following her strokes, "I was angry at the whole world, including God. I skipped denial and went straight to anger." But something had changed since that previous interview. This time, she spoke cheerfully of the prospect of her own death, saying she had been praying to die ever since the strokes had incapacitated her. Her advice for those who want to die well: Live well. "I always say that death can be one of the greatest experiences ever. If you have lived each day of your life right, then you have nothing to fear. Live so you don't look back and regret that you've wasted your life. Live life honestly and full," she said.[7]

Having moved through her anger to a place of acceptance, Elisabeth Kübler-Ross found a new perspective on her suffering. Life, she believes, is for learning, and God will give you what you need in order to learn, even—paradoxically—a ruptured blood vessel in the brain. "When you have learned all you have come to learn and taught all the things you can teach, then you can graduate to the next level," she says. "You may not get what you want, but God always gives you what you need."[8]

One foot in eternity

How do we get past our fear of death? The answer to that question is threefold:

1. *Don't avoid the issue.* Face death squarely, and accept death for what it is: the end of your mortal existence.

2. *Live well so you can die well.* Become the kind of person in life that you would want to be in death.

3. *Get in touch with the Infinite.* Connect your soul to the eternal.

If you develop your spirituality throughout your life, you will be more at ease with your mortality as death approaches. But if you only take out your spiritual beliefs and dust them off when you are in the valley of the shadow of death, it may be too late. The reality of death should cause us to focus daily on the reality of life. Every single day of our lives, we should be lining our souls with courage, confidence, and character in preparation for the day when we will need them the most. If we live our lives with one foot already in eternity, it won't be so hard to place the other foot there when the time comes.

So let your soul rattle loose in your body. Lean out into eternity. When your time comes to leave this planet, spread your arms like wings and sail toward home.

Questioning the Infinite

Does God Exist?

Gene Roddenberry, the creator of *Star Trek*, was a confirmed atheist. I never met him, but my good friend, actress Grace Lee Whitney, knew him well. "I first met Gene in 1963," Grace told me, "when he put me in an episode of his TV series *The Lieutenant*, with Gary Lockwood and Robert Vaughn. He remembered my work in that show and cast me in the pilot for another series called *Police Story*, with DeForest Kelley. *Police Story* didn't sell, but Gene plucked DeForest and me from that pilot and put us in his new science-fiction series, *Star Trek*.

"I remember many philosophical conversations I had with Gene in the studio commissary or in his office during the spring and summer of 1966, as *Star Trek* was moving into production. We talked a lot about the show—but we also talked about politics and social issues, about equality between the sexes, and about our shared atheist convictions. I was a Jewish atheist at the time—I loved the traditions of Judaism but I had no faith in God."

Halfway through the first season of *Star Trek*, Grace was sexually assaulted by a studio executive and subsequently fired from the series. That devastating event triggered a disastrous slide into alcoholism, drug addiction, and sex addiction that nearly killed her. Grace's salvation came in the form of a Twelve Step recovery program—a spiritual program in which she found sobriety through dependence upon a Power greater than herself.

Gene Roddenberry, by contrast, remained an atheist until his death in October 1991. Raised by a devout Southern Baptist mother and a father who openly scoffed at religion, Roddenberry became a confirmed atheist by his early teens. In an interview with *The Humanist*, published shortly before his death, he recalled:

In my early teens, I decided to listen to the sermon. I guess I was around fourteen and emerging as a personality. I had never really paid much attention to the sermon before. I was more interested in the deacon's daughter and what we might be doing between services.

I listened to the sermon, and I remember complete astonishment because what they were talking about were things that were just crazy....I guess from that time it was clear to me that religion was largely nonsense—largely magical, superstitious things. In my own teen life, I just couldn't see any point in adopting something based on magic, which was obviously phony and superstitious.[1]

Gene Roddenberry saw belief in God as illogical and unscientific. Atheism, he believed, was the enlightened, scientific world view. But as you are about to discover, Roddenberry was tragically mistaken.

Squirming with revulsion

Dr. George Greenstein is a Yale-educated astrophysicist. Some years ago, he became attracted to a concept called "the anthropic principle," which was first formulated by physicist Brandon Carter. "Anthropic" comes from the Greek word *anthropos*, meaning "man." The anthropic principle has to do with the conditions necessary for human beings to exist in the universe. Carter had noticed that a large number of unrelated laws of physics appeared to be coordinated, fine-tuned, and delicately balanced to produce life—almost as if the universe had been intelligently engineered by a Godlike superbeing. A confirmed atheist, Greenstein began examining the list of these "coincidental" conditions purely as a matter of personal amusement.

He started with a list he had jotted on a scrap of notebook paper. But as he kept reading scholarly papers by Carter and other scientists, his list kept growing. Soon, he had filled several pages of a notebook with anthropic "coincidences"—and the results were disturbing. "The more I read," he relates in his book *The Symbiotic Universe*, "the more I became convinced that such 'coincidences' could hardly have happened by chance." In other words, these anthropic "coincidences" began to look like evidence for a Cosmic Designer—evidence for *God*. Many people would consider scientific evidence for God to be *good* news. Not Greenstein. Instead, he says he experienced "an intense revulsion, and at times it was almost physical in nature. I would positively squirm with discomfort...I found it difficult to entertain the notion without grimacing in disgust, and well-nigh impossible to mention it to friends without apology."[2]

The possibility that God or a Godlike superbeing might have actually created the universe made Greenstein almost physically sick. Using vivid terms like "intense revulsion," "squirm with discomfort," and "grimacing in disgust," he frankly acknowledges his strong emotional bias against the God hypothesis. I applaud his candor.

I first encountered the anthropic principle in the April 1987 issue of *Analog Science Fiction/Science Fact*. Sandwiched among the science fiction stories was a fact article by Richard D. Meisner with the intriguing title "Universe—the Ultimate Artifact?" I began reading—and what I read was startling. In that article, Meisner checked off the same laundry list of cosmic "coincidences" that so appalled and repelled Greenstein. Meisner's conclusion: According to the scientific evidence, the universe appears to be an *artifact*—an object designed by an intelligent entity for an intelligent purpose. Meisner went on to quote several distinguished scientists—and what they said made them sound more like theologians than scientists. Astronomer Sir Fred Hoyle:

> A commonsense interpretation of the facts suggests that a super-intellect has monkeyed with physics, as well as chemistry and biology, and that there are no blind forces worth speaking about in nature.

And cosmologist Paul Davies:

> It is hard to resist the impression that the present structure of the universe, apparently so sensitive to minor alterations in the numbers, has been rather carefully thought out.

Then Meisner offered his own impression:

> One may feel inclined to apply the word "God" in this context. This is justifiable, although I tend to avoid the word simply because I've found almost without exception that it triggers an

immediate positive or negative emotional response in the listener—most inconducive to good scientific thinking. Naturally, the artifact hypothesis is most attractive when stripped of its unfortunate historical trappings of superstition and dogma....Personally, if the artifact inference proved true, I would be most interested not in *how* the universe was fabricated, but *why*.[3]

Why a universe? Why life? We'll get to these questions—but first, let's look at the evidence that made George Greenstein "squirm with discomfort."

The creative blast

The universe began with a bang.

The term "Big Bang" was actually coined by an opponent of the theory—astronomer Sir Fred Hoyle. During a radio talk over the BBC in 1950, Hoyle derisively referred to what he called "this Big Bang idea." To Hoyle's dismay, the term was enthusiastically adopted by supporters of the Big Bang theory. Today, there is no doubt among physicists that the Big Bang truly did happen some fifteen billion years ago. Thanks to measurements made by space-based telescopes and high energy particle accelerators, scientists have a very good understanding of the evolution of the universe from the first trillionth of a second to the present day.

In 1992, a team of astrophysicists tabulated over four hundred million temperature measurements collected by NASA's Cosmic Background Explorer (COBE). In the process, they discovered faint fluctuations in the background microwave radiation of the universe—the lingering echo of the Big Bang. These fluctuations—"ripples in the fabric of spacetime," as they were called by research director George Smoot (astrophysicist, U.C. Berkeley)—explain how galaxies formed and clustered together out of the initially smooth and uniform Big Bang. Smoot said, "It's like looking at God," and cosmologist Steven Hawking called the COBE findings "the discovery of the century, if not of all time."[4]

What many people don't realize is that the Big Bang is not something that happened billions of years ago. It is still happening now. The universe is still expanding, and we are living inside the most massive explosion there ever was. The sheer size and force of the Big Bang aside, this was no ordinary explosion, in which material was blasted outwards into empty space. Rather, the Big Bang actually *created* space and time. At the beginning of the Big Bang, everything that is—matter, energy, the three dimensions of space, and the fourth dimension of time—blossomed forth from a single geometric point, swelling at the speed of light.

Physicists and cosmologists are amazed that such a violent event as the Big Bang could have been so delicately balanced. In *God and the New Physics*, Paul Davies observes

> Had the Big Bang been weaker, the cosmos would have soon fallen back on itself in a big crunch. On the other hand, had it been stronger, the cosmic material would have dispersed so rapidly that galaxies would not have formed....Had the explosion differed in strength at the outset by only one part in 10^{60}, the universe we now perceive would not exist. To give some meaning to these numbers, suppose you wanted to fire a bullet at a one-inch target on the other side of the observable universe, twenty billion light-years away. Your aim would have to be accurate to that same part in 10^{60}....
>
> Channeling the explosive violence into such a regular and organized pattern of motion seems like a miracle.[5]

When you add all the other anthropic coincidences (which we will examine shortly) to the seeming "miracle" of the Big Bang, the universe looks even less like a random accident. As Roger Penrose, Rouse Ball Professor of Mathematics at Oxford, observes in *The Emperor's New Mind*:

> The Creator's aim must have been...to an accuracy of
>
> $$\text{one part in } 10^{10^{10^{123}}}$$

> This is an extraordinary figure. One could not possibly even *write the number down* in full, in the ordinary denary notation: it would be '1' followed by 10^{123} successive '0's! Even if we were to write a '0' on each separate proton and on each separate neutron in the entire universe—and we could throw in all the other particles as well for good measure—we should fall far short of writing down the figure needed.[6]

Creation was perfectly balanced. It was adjusted and fine-tuned to a tolerance of practically one part in infinity. Had the Big Bang not been so delicately balanced, concludes George Greenstein, "the cosmos would have winked out of existence the instant after it had been created."[7]

Creation was a blast. A *perfect* blast. It gives every appearance of having been flawlessly engineered by some cosmic Master Blaster.

Deep space and deep time

In 1972, Nobel-winning French biologist Jacques Monod published an influential book, *Chance and Necessity*, in which he stated, "Man knows at last that he is alone in the universe's unfeeling immensity, out of which he emerged only by chance." A grim conclusion? Certainly. But it is merely the *logical* conclusion of a trend that began in 1514, when a Polish priest named Nicholas Copernicus first suggested that the Earth is *not* the center of the universe. The result of the so-called "Copernican revolution" has been to steadily shrink human significance under a crushing weight of infinite time and infinite space.

But the evidence of the anthropic principle has shown Monod to be wrong—and has completely reversed the Copernican revolution. Yes, the universe is incomprehensibly vast and ancient—but that doesn't mean human life is insignificant. Far from it.

To get an idea of the enormity of the cosmic scale, consider this analogy: At the end of this sentence is a period. Let that period represent Planet Earth. Now, let's say you lay eleven copies of this book end to end. (In fact, why don't you go out to the bookstore right now and buy ten more copies of this book and try it yourself? I'll wait here till you get back.) Okay, you have your eleven copies of this book laid end-to-end? Good. That is the distance from the Sun to Planet Earth (represented by that period). And how big is the Sun? According to this scale, the diameter of the Sun is roughly the thickness of this book. Now, how far is the nearest star system, Alpha Centauri? To find out, you would have to get in your car and drive about four hundred miles.

In the full-scale universe, Alpha Centauri is a triple star group a mere 4.2 light-years from your doorstep. And what about the other stars in our general neighborhood? Well, the star Altair (where Leslie Nielsen fell head over heels for Anne Francis in the movie *Forbidden Planet*) is 16.5 light-years away. The star Antares is about 500-some-odd light-years away; so is Betelgeuse, though in a different direction. Rigel is way the heck out there—around 900 light-years away. But in astronomical terms, all of these stars are actually right in our own cozy little suburb of the Milky Way.

Our Milky Way galaxy is a big place—a spiral-shaped collection of some one hundred billion stars. It measures some one hundred thousand light-years in diameter. In our corner of the galaxy, stars are spaced an average of thirty trillion miles apart. It takes our solar system about two hundred million years to make one trip all the way around the galaxy. And our galaxy is only one of one hundred billion galaxies scattered in clusters across a trillion-trillion cubic light-years of empty, meaningless, "wasted" space.

With that as our perspective, we can see that we stand on the shore of our little backwater world, circling a third-rate star at the outer edge of just one galaxy out of swarms and swarms of galaxies. So who do we think we are? Who are we that the universe is mindful of us? We are insignificant flyspecks living meaningless lives on a transitory dust mote, right?

Wrong.

The immensity of time and the immensity of space should not make us feel small and insignificant. All of that vast, mind-numbing space-time literally makes our lives possible. It nurtures us and keeps us safe. It is just one more piece of evidence to suggest that *our universe was designed to produce intelligent life.* As Richard Meisner observes, "The overwhelming size, age, and emptiness of the universe, far from being indications of the insignificance of intelligent life, are in fact prerequisites for the existence of such life."[8] All that "wasted space" is not wasted at all. The universe had to be that big, that old, and that empty so that you and I could exist.

Just look at what had to take place in order for intelligent life to arise on this little dust mote of ours. First, galaxies had to form—that process took the first few billion years of cosmic history. The first generation of stars were made of hydrogen and helium—there were no heavier elements anywhere in the universe. All the heavier elements, such as carbon, nitrogen, and oxygen, had to be cooked up in the hearts of stars over several billion years.

An entire generation of stars had to be born, live, and die in order to create these heavier elements. Then those stars had to explode and scatter their elements into space, forming planets. Our own Earth has only been around for about a third of the age of the universe, and humanity has only been around for a fraction of 1 percent of the age of the earth. It took the universe a long time to produce the human race.

But that is how the laws of physics work: The universe *had to be* this big and this old for intelligent life to arise. People like us (or even alien beings such as Vulcans, Romulans, or Klingons) just couldn't have arrived on the scene much sooner than we did. The raw materials needed to make people didn't exist for the first few billion years of cosmic existence. I don't care what birth date you put down on your driver's license, it took around fifteen billion years to make one *you*. (Hey, you can't rush perfection, right?) So the thought of all that time and all that space shouldn't make you feel "alone in the universe's unfeeling immensity." It should make you feel pretty special.

If you've seen one of those killer asteroid movies like *Armageddon* or *Deep Impact*, then you already know another important reason for the mind-boggling emptiness of space: Vast space is our security blanket. It reduces the odds of collisions with asteroids, comets, planets, stars, and black holes. Near the core of our galaxy, where the star population is much denser and there is far less empty space, stars collide with stars, planet orbits are unstable, and black holes gobble up anything in reach. Not a nice neighborhood to live in. Scientists are convinced that life could not arise and survive near the center of the galaxy.

So be glad you were born on the outskirts of the Milky Way. It may not be as uptown as the galactic core, but it's home.

The carbon connection

You need carbon to make diamonds, pencil leads, petroleum, and people. You even need carbon to make alien life forms. As Richard Meisner observes, the most exotic alien imaginable (even one which would use, say, liquid ammonia instead of water in its cells and bloodstream) "still requires carbon in its alternate forms of fats, lipids, amino acids, carbohydrates, proteins, and nucleic acids."[9] Fortunately, there is plenty of carbon in the universe—but why? For decades, scientists pondered the fact that *carbon should not exist*. As it turns out, the creation of carbon depends on another delicately balanced condition in the laws of physics.

The problem that confronted physicists was that there was no known mechanism by which three helium nuclei could simultaneously collide inside a star and fuse to form a carbon nucleus. In 1952, American astrophysicist Ed Salpeter suggested that perhaps carbon was formed in a rapid two-step process: two helium nuclei could collide, forming an unstable beryllium nucleus—so unstable, in fact, that it could only exist for less than a trillionth of a second. During that trillionth of a second, a third helium nucleus *just might* collide with the beryllium nucleus and form a carbon nucleus. It quickly became clear, however, that this process would yield little if any carbon, since the unstable beryllium nucleus was more likely to be split by, instead of fusing with, the third helium nucleus.

Then English astronomer Fred Hoyle entered the fray. He took Salpeter's idea and added a new wrinkle: *nuclear resonance*. The nucleus of an atom can exist in a number of discrete states, depending on its energy level. Expose that nucleus to a given amount of energy and it will *resonate* at a specific frequency. This resonance makes it much easier for atoms to fuse and form new elements.

Hoyle reasoned that, since carbon clearly *does* exist in abundance (if it didn't, we would not exist), then carbon *must* have been created in a resonant reaction. So much carbon could never have been created by nonresonant processes. So, knowing that the energy level of helium and beryllium in the high-temperature conditions inside a star was about 7.4 million electron volts (MeV), Hoyle predicted there *must* be an unknown resonance level for carbon waiting to be discovered—a level just above 7.4 MeV.

Hoyle urged his physicist buddies to perform the experiment, using a particle accelerator. "Fred," they scoffed, "we already know all the resonance levels for carbon. The one you want just ain't there." Hoyle smiled. "Humor me," he said. So they conducted the experiment—and Hoyle was right. The resonance level was right where Hoyle predicted: 7.65 MeV.

Hoyle's finding is significant in a number of ways: This resonance level is very precisely adjusted to allow for the production of life-giving carbon. Anything other than the precise level of 7.65 MeV would render carbon nonexistent, or a rare trace element at best. Life would be impossible.

There is another resonance level for the production of oxygen—but fortunately, the resonance level for oxygen is *just 1 percent less* than the resonance level of a helium-plus-carbon reaction (helium and carbon are used to make oxygen). That tiny 1 percent misadjustment is just enough to prevent all of that beautiful life-giving carbon from—*poof!*—transmuting into oxygen. Fortunately, stars manufacture all the oxygen we need through nonresonant reactions alone—but if not for that tiny 1 percent of misadjustment, oxygen production would have run wild and all carbon in the universe would have quickly disappeared.

The instability of the beryllium nucleus is also precisely adjusted; it decays in just 1/1,000,000,000,000,000 second—and this helps to slow down the fusion process inside a star. If the beryllium nucleus were slightly more stable, fusion of heavier elements would proceed so rapidly that the star would explode too soon, before enough of these elements had been created. If the beryllium nucleus were slightly less stable, carbon and other heavier elements would never form.

As Richard Meisner observes, "The advantageous placement of these resonance levels are necessary and finely-tuned conditions for the existence of life in this universe."[10] And George Greenstein agrees. "It's hard to see why those nuclei should work together so smoothly," he notes. "Others do not. Other nuclear reactions do not proceed by such a remarkable chain of lucky breaks....Why should such disparate structures [as helium, beryllium, and carbon] mesh together so perfectly? Upon this wildly unlikely coincidence our existence, and that of every life form in the universe, depends."[11]

Hoyle's discovery is significant because he actually devised a testable hypothesis that affirms the validity of the anthropic principle. He realized that in order for human beings to exist, the resonance level for carbon *had to be* located at a specific energy level, and he predicted precisely where that energy level would be found. In other words, *Fred Hoyle had to think one of the Creator's own thoughts* in order to solve the mystery of carbon.

The cosmic conspiracy

The list of cosmic coincidences goes on and on. It is as if dozens of wildly unrelated laws of nature plotted together in a cosmic conspiracy to produce life. Individually, each of these laws is a deal-breaker. If *just one* of these conditions were not perfectly fine-tuned and precisely balanced, life would be impossible. Some examples:

There are four forces governing the microrealm of subatomic particles—the electromagnetic force, the gravitational force, the "strong" nuclear force and the "weak" nuclear force. These forces determine the structure of the universe, from how an electron orbits the nucleus of an atom to how Planet Earth stays in orbit around the Sun. Each of these forces has a specific mathematical value called a *constant*—so-called because that value never varies.

At first, the constants were simply accepted as a brute fact—no one wondered why this or that constant was not 1 percent stronger or weaker than it is. Eventually, physicists and cosmologists began to realize that the laws of the universe were encoded into the structure of the universe at the moment of the Big Bang. As George Greenstein observes, "The laws of nature could have been laid down only in the very instant of the creation of the universe, if not before."[12] As scientists discovered that the laws of nature might have been different than they are, they began to look at those constants with new awe and respect. Here are some of the fine-tuned physical constants they discovered:

The gravitational force constant was finely tuned to permit life. Slightly greater, and stars would burn too hot, too quickly, and too unevenly. Slightly smaller, and stars would be too cool, so that nuclear fusion could not take place and there would be no life-giving heavier elements. The electromagnetic force is also fine-tuned—if its constant was slightly larger or smaller, the chemical bonding required for making living things could not take place. There is also a delicate balance between the gravitational and electromagnetic forces. If the constant of the ratio between these two forces were larger, there would be no stars smaller than 1.4 solar masses, and the lifetime of stars would be short; if the constant were smaller, there would be no stars larger than 0.8 solar masses—and no production of life-giving heavier elements.

If the strong nuclear force constant were slightly larger, there would be no hydrogen in the universe and no stars; smaller, and the universe would be nothing *but* hydrogen. If the weak force constant were larger, most of the hydrogen in the universe would have converted to helium during the Big Bang; smaller, and there would be too little hydrogen converted to helium—a roadblock to the production of life-giving heavier elements such as carbon and oxygen.

A proton is 1,836 times more massive than an electron; if this ratio varied slightly in either direction, molecules could not form and life could not exist. The ratio of the number of protons to the number of electrons is finely balanced to permit the electromagnetic force to dominate the gravitational force, allowing the formation of galaxies, stars, and planets. The expansion rate of the universe is finely balanced to permit the formation of stars and galaxies. And the list goes on: the proton decay rate, the mass inequality between the neutron and proton, the matter-antimatter ratio, and more—so many fine-tuned, interlocking, precision-aligned conditions, all focused on producing life, all laid down at the moment of Creation. It becomes hard to view the universe we live in as a random toss of the cosmic dice.

"As we survey all the evidence," George Greenstein reflects in *The Symbiotic Universe*, "the thought insistently arises that some supernatural agency—or, rather, Agency—must be involved. Is it possible that suddenly, without intending to, we have stumbled upon scientific proof of the existence of a Supreme Being?"[13] Greenstein's answer to his own question: No. But his rejection of the God hypothesis, he freely admits, is not based on any evidence. It is based purely on personal preference. "It is a matter of taste how one deals with [the notion of God]," he writes. "Those who wish are free to accept it, and I have no way to prove them wrong. But I know where I stand....I reject it utterly. I will have nothing to do with it."[14]

Having rejected the God hypothesis as an explanation for the anthropic coincidences, how does Greenstein explain them? Well, he envisions a universe that mysteriously "bootstraps" itself into existence through a symbiotic relationship between the cosmos and intelligent life. In other words, he claims that the universe needs intelligent life in order to become "real," and intelligent life needs a universe in which to live—*so the universe and life mutually bring each other into existence*. He is understandably vague on exactly how that works.

Why does Greenstein concoct such a counterintuitive (one is tempted to say "illogical") scenario to account for the anthropic evidence? On the face of it, the evidence clearly suggests the work of an intelligent Cosmic Designer. Why, then, does Greenstein reject the God hypothesis out of hand? Answer: The problem of evil. Greenstein reasons that an all-good, all-powerful God would never allow the evil and suffering we see in our world. Hence God does not exist.

As we have seen earlier in this book, Greenstein is not alone. Many people find the problem of evil to be a major roadblock to belief in God. For other people, there are different roadblocks. Some reject belief in God because they have been mistreated or exploited by people who claim to speak for God. Others consider the idea of God laughable because of the ridiculous stereotypes projected by televangelists and faith healers. Still others simply have a problem with authority—*any* authority—and since God represents the Ultimate Authority in the universe, they have a *big* problem with God. These are, of course, emotional rather than rational reasons for rejecting the God hypothesis—but emotional arguments can be extremely persuasive.

In *Human Society in Ethics and Politics,* Bertrand Russell observed, "There is something feeble and a little contemptible about a man who cannot face the perils of life without the help of comfortable myths." By "comfortable myths," of course, he means belief in God. Skeptics like Russell see faith as a superstitious "crutch" for people who cannot face the reality of a godless, meaningless universe. Well, it's certainly true that believers find the reality of God a comforting idea. But atheism, too, can be a "comfortable myth," a "crutch." There are those, like George Greenstein, who squirm with revulsion, discomfort, and disgust at the chilling notion of a Cosmic Authority. So rather than face the reality of God's existence, they retreat from the evidence of the anthropic principle and seek refuge in the "comfortable myth" of atheism.

Emotion and personal preference are hardly reliable guides to a realistic worldview. We can't wish God *into* existence simply because we can't face living in a meaningless world. Nor can we wish God *out of* existence simply because we don't like the idea of an Ultimate Authority. Regardless of what we *wish* to be true, regardless of our biases, regardless of our discomfort, there is an *objective* truth to be determined. There either is a God or there isn't. That's reality. We owe it to ourselves to follow the evidence wherever it leads, and to live courageously, realistically, and rationally, in accordance with the way the world really *is*.

Who or what Is God?

I don't believe people squirm with discomfort over the *reality* of God. They squirm with discomfort over their *flawed mental conceptions* of God. The reason there are so many agnostics and atheists in the world is that there are so many corrosive stereotypes of God in the world. These stereotypes prevent people from discovering the *reality* of God.

We human beings have a tendency to reduce God to metaphors and images. Such conceptions of God can be comforting (Father, Patriarch, Mother, Provider, Friend, Guide, Shepherd, Benevolent Ruler). Or they can be disturbing (Cruel Judge or Capricious Fate or Unfeeling Cosmic Immensity). Many people superimpose a mental image of their parents over their image of God. These images can sometimes be painful and destructive, as when victims of a dysfunctional childhood imagine God as an absent, rejecting, or abusive parent. But metaphors and images are symbols, not reality.

Some conceptions of God are downright silly, such as the classic conception of a bearded old man in the long white robe. In this book, I have tried to avoid anthropomorphic stereotypes of God. I have even avoided, for the most part, any pronouns for God, since English personal pronouns always reflect gender. To call God "He" or "She" would, in my mind, limit God to the status of an anthropomorphic god or goddess. There is no scientific evidence that God possesses gender (though, if human beings are created in the image of God, as the world's great religions attest, then God's nature must encompass the intellectual/emotional attributes of *both* masculinity and femininity).

Some people, in an attempt to shed all metaphors and images of God, are left with a mental image of a great Nothing. But God is not nothing. True, God is *no thing*—that is, the God of the anthropic evidence has an existence that is not bound to the created realm of *things*. A God that stands outside of time and space, a God that can design the structure of the universe and shape the explosive forces of the Big Bang, is *no thing*, but is certainly not nothing. A God that is an infinite Nothingness is a mere abstraction. Our universe was not designed by an abstraction. Moreover, we cannot relate to an abstraction. If our conception of God is one of murkiness and nothingness, then our conception is flawed and unreal.

So what is the reality of God? What can we truly know about God? Here is what the evidence of the anthropic principle tells us about God:

- God is real.

- God is intelligent and purposeful.

• Because God is intelligent and purposeful, God is a *self*, not just a "force" or a "principle."

• God is able to design and create a universe of perfectly balanced laws and conditions.

• God is interested in life—particularly intelligent life.

• God is transcendent—that is, God is above, beyond, and prior to the laws of nature (and thus, presumably, not bound by those laws).

Notice, please, that there is one thing I did *not* say about God. I did not say that God is a "supernatural" being. The anthropic evidence says nothing about the "supernatural."

The stereotype of God as a "supernatural" being is, I think, one of the great barriers that keeps many people from believing in God. To some, the word *supernatural* suggests creatures of myth and fantasy, such as ghosts, werewolves, vampires, and witches. A "supernatural" realm is one in which the laws of science, reason, and logic no longer apply. It is a realm where our intelligence is insulted and assaulted and rendered meaningless, a place where reality is up for grabs, where anything can and does happen, for no good reason and with no sensible explanation. If God is a "supernatural" being, then God is an irrational being who violates his own laws on a whim.

It is this view of God as an irrational, "supernatural" being that leads physicist George Greenstein to say, "I reject the supernatural."[15] In the same way, *Star Trek* producer Gene Roddenberry complained of being raised in a family that believed in a "supernatural" God—a God who makes no rational sense. As he told one interviewer:

I was born into a supernatural world in which all my people—my family—usually said, "That is because God willed it," or gave other supernatural explanations for whatever happened. When you confront those statements on their own, they just don't make sense. They are clearly wrong. You need a certain amount of proof to accept anything, and that proof was not forthcoming to support those statements.[16]

Well, the image of God that emerges from the anthropic evidence is a God that *does* make sense. There is nothing supernatural about the anthropic principle. In fact, the anthropic evidence presents us with a universe that is rational, orderly, and purposeful. If, as the evidence suggests, there truly is an intelligent Cosmic Designer, then that Designer seems to have arranged for human beings to be able to think and reason. This is a key insight, because it is our *God-given intelligence* that is offended by irrational concepts of a "supernatural" realm.

Thinking people cannot accept the idea of a God who is arbitrary, irrational, and capricious. And the evidence of the anthropic principle shows that the Cosmic Designer is anything but.

The God hypothesis

The French astronomer, the Marquis de Laplace (1749–1827), presented a copy of his *Celestial Mechanics* to Emperor Napoleon Bonaparte. Napoleon read the book from cover to cover, then sent for Laplace and said, "You have written a very large book about the universe. Yet nowhere in this book do you mention the Author of the universe."

"Sire," Laplace replied, "I had no need of that hypothesis."

Today, the God hypothesis is not only needed—the evidence seems to demand it. I am convinced that the Author of the universe has given us an artifact that proves *God is*. We can't ignore that artifact, because we are living in it. It surrounds and nurtures us. It is our home, our universe, our time-and-space reality. If we are to live rationally and realistically, then we have to deal with the truth that confronts us.

Many people are able to just *know* and *trust* in God's reality, without needing to see the scientific evidence. But others ask, "How can I believe in the reality of Something for which there is no evidence?" The good news for those who have been plagued by questions and doubts is that the scientific evidence is now pouring in. To me, the anthropic evidence seems compelling, convincing—even satisfying. It confirms the observation of the thirteenth century German mystic, Meister Eckhardt, who said, "God is like a person who clears his throat while hiding and so gives himself away." At times, God does indeed seem to hide—but if you listen carefully, you can hear an unmistakable "ahem!" echoing through the cosmos.

I remember one night, when I was seven or eight years old, I was in bed, lying awake, wondering about God. An idea came to me: If God is really God, then it should be no problem for the Creator to arrange a convincing demonstration. A loving God would surely be willing to do that for a little kid, right? So I prayed, "God, if you are real, then prove it. Pick up that ball and make it hover around the room. If you can't do just one little thing to prove you are real, then I'll never believe in you again."

I waited and I watched the ball. It didn't rise off the floor. It didn't hover. It didn't even budge. "Well...?" I prompted.

Both God and the ball remained stubbornly unmoved. I waited...

"Okay," I said to the darkness, "we'll talk about this later."

I didn't realize it or understand it at the time, but God was answering my prayer (though it was really more of a dare than a prayer). God didn't answer in the way I wanted, of course—and God certainly didn't answer according to my timetable. God waited a few decades, then came up with something much better and more convincing than a cheap parlor trick like a levitating ball. God used the whole universe to announce, "Here I am." I'm glad I was around to hear it.

Today, I am convinced beyond a reasonable doubt. The question "Does God exist?" has been asked and answered. The answer is a rational one, grounded in scientific evidence. I don't know if this answer satisfies your soul or not, but I know it satisfies mine.

In case you are *not* fully satisfied, just turn the page. There are more and deeper answers still to come....

17

What Is the Soul?

Kim Alexis is not only a supermodel, but a super athlete as well. Her running coach, a man named Hank, encouraged her to run marathons. At first, Kim thought Hank was kidding. A marathon is a grueling endurance test—a cross-country race more than twenty-six miles long. But Hank persuaded her to try. Kim ran her first marathon in Jacksonville, Florida, and Hank ran beside her the entire race, holding her hand as they crossed the finish line. It was the first of several marathons she participated in, with Hank's coaching.

Hank was not just Kim's coach. He was a friend. About ten years into their friendship, Hank was diagnosed with cancer. He underwent treatment and the cancer went into remission for a time—but it returned.

The last time Kim saw Hank face-to-face was in May 1995. Kim and her husband Ron were in Florida for a charity event. They met Hank and his wife Jody for dinner at a restaurant. "At one point," Kim told me, "Hank leaned over and said, 'Kim, it's all through me.' That's all he said about the cancer. It was like he wanted me to know it was serious—but he refused to dwell on the negative. The next moment, he was talking and joking like he didn't have a care in the world."

"How old was he?" I asked.

"Fifty," Kim replied, "and he looked healthy. But over the next few months, the cancer just ravaged him. His weight dropped to ninety pounds and he couldn't even walk. But he never believed he was going to die. I called Hank and Jody a number of times—they lived in Arkansas—and he'd always say, 'I can't wait to beat this thing so I can get out and run again.'"

But Hank would never run again.

Shortly before Christmas 1995, Kim went to a studio in Los Angeles to record some radio spots. "A studio sound booth is very quiet," she told me, "like a prayer chapel. I had about twenty scripts to read, and while I was recording the spots, I suddenly had the strangest feeling. I had a strong impression that Hank was in the sound booth with me, standing behind me. The feeling was so strong I turned around to see if he were there."

"Was it just a feeling that *someone* was in the booth with you?" I asked. "Or was it specifically Hank?"

"Oh, definitely Hank," she replied. "I knew it was him."

"How long did that sense of Hank's presence last?"

She paused. "At least ten minutes," she replied. "Maybe fifteen. I finished the taping—it took about an hour. As soon as I got out of the booth, I called my husband. I said, 'Ron, is there something going on with Hank? I just had the strangest feeling about him.' He said, 'Jody just called. Hank died about an hour ago.' And that was just when I had sensed his presence. I don't know how these things work, but I believe he came to tell me good-bye, because we'd been such good friends."

Kim's experience is not *scientific* proof of the reality of the soul, of course, but it is difficult to discount or dismiss. And there is a good deal more evidence to indicate the reality of the immortal human soul. I believe the soul is real—not because I wish it were so, but because that's where the evidence leads.

Body and soul

What do we mean by the word *soul*? Today, people generally use *soul* interchangeably with the word *spirit*. In *Denial of the Soul*, for example, M. Scott Peck defines the soul as "a God-created, God-nurtured, unique, developable, immortal human spirit."[1]

In ancient times, however, the soul was seen as distinct from the spirit. The Hebrews saw the nonmaterial component of a human being as consisting of the soul (*nephesh*) and the spirit (*ruwach*). The ancient Greeks, too, made a distinction between soul and spirit. The Greek word for soul was *psuche*, from which we get the word *psychology*—the study of the soul. The soul or *psuche* is the force of life and the seat of the mind, will, emotions, and conscience. The Greek word for spirit was *pneuma*, a word which suggested breath or wind. The *pneuma* was thought to depart the body at death and could not be dissolved by death.

For our purposes, let's simply define the soul as the essential, eternal I-ness—the indestructible and immortal core of our being. The soul, let us say, is that which lives on after the death of the body.

Of course, not everyone agrees that the soul exists. Those who do not believe in the soul hold the *monist* view—the belief that the material world is all there is to reality. The monist sees consciousness as merely a temporary function of the brain. When the body dies, the mind disappears—end of story. Science fiction writer Isaac Asimov typified this view when he wrote:

> The molecules of my body, after my conception, added other molecules and arranged the whole into more and more complex form....In the process, I developed, little by little, into a conscious something I call "I" that exists only as the arrangement. When the arrangement is lost forever, as it will be when I die, the "I" will be lost forever, too.
>
> And that suits me fine. No concept I have ever heard, of either a Hell or of a Heaven, has seemed to me to be suitable for a civilized rational mind to inhabit, and I would rather have the nothingness.[2]

In contrast to the monist view is the *dualist* view, the belief that mind and matter are two fundamentally different substances. According to this view, the soul is only temporarily contained by the material body. The body dies, but the soul continues on—either moving on to Heaven or Hell (as in Christianity), or returning via reincarnation (as in Eastern religion). There is an intrinsic relationship between body and soul, mortality and immortality. The body gives form and visible expression to the soul, as Walt Whitman suggests in "I Sing the Body Electric":

> O I say these are not the parts and poems of the body only,
> but of the soul,
> O I say now these are the soul!

The quantum and the soul

The branch of physics that studies the structure and behavior of atoms and subatomic particles is called quantum mechanics. The QM realm may seem an odd place to go soul-searching, but it is there that we find compelling scientific evidence that the soul is real.

The quantum world is spooky and weird. It does not behave as you would expect. An atom, for example, is composed of a nucleus orbited by a whirling cloud of electrons. The location of an electron orbit is rigidly defined by a famous law of physics called the inverse square law. An electron orbiting a nucleus can *only* be found in one of those precisely defined orbits, and the energy of the electron determines which orbit it is in. If you change the energy of an electron, it will change orbits—but in a way that totally violates common sense. It does not *move* from one orbit to the next—it winks out *here* and reappears *there*—the so-called "quantum leap."

How is it possible for an electron to disappear in one place and reappear in another? Because an electron is not a *thing*. It is *real*—but it has *no substance*. Hang in. It gets stranger still.

Scientists have conducted experiments with electrons and photons to determine just what they are. In one kind of experiment, these entities behave as particles like tiny little bullets. But in another kind of experiment, they don't behave like particles at all. They behave like waves. Scientists call this dual nature of QM entities "wave-particle duality." Physicist Jean-Marc Lévy-Leblond suggests that such entities be called "partiqles" (with a "q" for quantum replacing the "c" in "particle") to make it clear that a quantum partiqle is *not* a solid object.

Partiqles do not "exist" in a common, everyday sense. The existence of a partiqle depends on the kind of experiment you perform on it. As physicist George Greenstein notes, "If someone is watching, the electron is a particle. If no one watches, it is a wave."[3] But this violates common sense! Certainly there is a *there* there, isn't there? How can we make a partiqle "real" simply by observing? Is this some kind of "mind over matter" thing? No, this is simple, everyday truth in the quantum realm. We don't make a partiqle "real" by willing it to be real, but simply by observing.

Quantum mechanics doesn't deal in certainties but in probabilities. The state of a quantum entity such as an atom or an electron can only be expressed by a mathematical equation called a *wave function*. The wave function of an electron describes all of its possible locations in space and time. Until the electron is observed and measured, it has no objective reality. It is a probability wave, a set of mathematical potentialities, a shimmering fleck of possibility waiting to exist. When an observer pokes the electron with his cloud chamber or other measuring device, the state of the electron is determined and becomes real. Scientists say that the act of observation *collapses the wave function* to a discrete state. This is why University of Texas physicist John Wheeler says we live in a "participatory universe." We participate with the quantum world in making reality real.

The strange implications of quantum mechanics are illustrated by the famous thought experiment called "Schrödinger's Cat" (after physicist Erwin Schrödinger). When I first explained this experiment to my daughter, she was horrified! "Oh, the poor kitty!" she protested. I explained to her that the experiment has never been performed with a live animal—only *hypothetical* cats are harmed in this experiment.

> "*I*f you change the energy of an electron, it will change orbits—but in a way that totally violates common sense. It does not move from one orbit to the next—it winks out here and reappears there—the so-called 'quantum leap.'"

Here's how it works: You seal a cat inside a box. In the box with the cat are a tiny quantity of radioactive material and a Geiger counter connected to a relay which, when activated, releases deadly cyanide gas inside the box. Over the space of an hour, there is a fifty-fifty chance that one atom in the radioactive material will decay. If an atom decays, the Geiger counter will detect it, trigger the relay, and cause the gas to be released, killing the cat. If an atom does not decay in an hour, the cat lives.

So you set up your fiendish little experiment and you wait. At the end of an hour, you wonder: Is the cat alive or dead? According to quantum mechanics, the cat is *neither*—and *both*. What you are measuring in this experiment is not merely the health of Schrödinger's cat but the state of an atom. Did it decay or not? The answer, so long as the box remains closed, can only be expressed as a wave function, a set of probabilities, not a certainty. And it's *not* simply because you don't know the answer yet. It's because *there is no real, objective reality until the observation is made.*

The wave function of both the atom and Schrödinger's cat is a fifty-fifty probability—what quantum physicists call a "superposition of states."

The atom exists in a decayed/non-decayed state and the cat exists in a dead/alive state—at the same time. And it gets weirder still.

Many quantum theorists hold a view called the Many-Worlds Interpretation (or MWI). According to MWI, the wave function does not collapse when you observe the cat. Instead, reality *fractures*. You and Schrödinger's cat and the entire universe split in two and follow two separate paths of reality. There is a dead cat reality and a live cat reality. The you that is in one reality is completely unaware of the you in the other reality.

Right now, at this very moment (according to the MWI), there are literally millions of yous following millions of paths of reality that have branched at every decision-point in your life. There are paths of reality in which you are married to a different mate, in which you are pursuing a different career, in which you are poor, rich, obscure, famous, living it up, and dead as a doornail. There are millions of realities in which you never existed. Each of these realities, according to the MWI, is as real as the reality in which you are holding this book in your hands and reading these words.

This mind-bending theory is responsible for a lot of "parallel universe" science fiction tales, such as Robert A. Heinlein's *Job: A Comedy of Justice* and Philip K. Dick's *The Man in the High Castle*. Science fiction writers love to ask what might have happened if Lincoln had survived the assassination attempt or if Hitler had won World War II. But it's not very pleasant to think that the close call you had on the freeway this morning might have actually killed you dead in an alternate reality.

Now, here is where the reality of God and the soul come in. Here is where we get to the heart of what I call Quantum Theology. Clearly, MWI produces a messy profusion of universes—literally trillions and trillions of universes. As physicist Paul Davies notes in *God and the New Physics*, "To invoke an infinity of other universes just to explain one is surely carrying excess baggage to cosmic extremes."[4] But this messy profusion of universes can be avoided if the wave function of *all reality* can be collapsed into a single discrete reality. I'm convinced this has already happened.

The quantum universe came into existence at the moment of the Big Bang. Yet, at that moment, intelligent observers (at least the only intelligent observers we know of—us!) would not evolve for another fifteen billion years. The Big Bang exploded and the universe expanded.

Galaxies, stars, and planets formed—yet not a single human being existed to observe it all.

But perhaps there was one observer. Perhaps the Cosmic *Designer* was also the Cosmic *Observer*. It may well be that, long before human beings arose, the Creator was observing the creation, collapsing the wave function of everything that is, creating objective reality out of quantum potentiality, making sure there would only be *one* you, not millions of yous.

And because you and I are intelligent observers, we now participate with the Cosmic Designer in shaping reality. We make observations and initiate actions that affect the universe. For some fifteen billion years, the Cosmic Designer collapsed the wave function of the universe without any help from anyone. But when we arrived on the scene, the Cosmic Designer gave us the ability to collapse the wave function of our own little corner of reality.

You may find it hard to believe that the universe could exist in a state of quantum uncertainty and unreality—but cosmologists and physicists don't find this hard to believe at all. Paul Davies writes in *The Mind of God*:

> Quantum mechanics, it will be recalled, incorporates Heisenberg's uncertainty principle, which has the effect of smearing out the values of all observable quantities in an unpredictable way. Thus an electron in orbit around an atom cannot be considered to have a well-defined position in space at every moment. One should not really think of it as circling the atomic nucleus along a definite path, but instead as smeared out in an indeterminate manner around the nucleus.
>
> Although this is the case for electrons in atoms, when it comes to macroscopic objects we do not observe such smearing. Thus the planet Mars has a definite position in space at each moment, and follows a definite orbit around the sun. In spite of this, Mars is still subject to the laws of quantum mechanics. One can now ask, as Enrico Fermi once did, why Mars is not smeared out around the sun in the same way as an electron is smeared out around an atom. In other words, given that the universe was born in a quantum event, how has an essentially non-quantum world emerged?[5]

Davies adds that physicists James Hartle and Murray Gell-Mann have calculated that the existence of our well-defined universe depends on finely tuned conditions at the beginning of the universe. According to their calculations, the real, discrete world we now inhabit is *statistically unlikely in the extreme*. This leads us to suspect that Something or Someone has collapsed the wave function for the entire universe, so that we now live in a distinct cosmos of distinct objects occupying definite locations in a clearly defined space-time.

Now, here is a crucial question: Why does the universe require *intelligent observers* in order to collapse a quantum wave function? Couldn't the wave function of a quantum particle collapse to a discrete state if it was merely detected by a Geiger counter or a cloud chamber? No. "The very cosmos does not exist unless observed," says George Greenstein, "And...*only a conscious mind is capable of performing such an observation....*Why do I claim that a conscious mind is required to bring it about? Why could an inanimate measuring instrument not do just as well?"[6]

Greenstein then explains what happens when an electron passes through a cloud chamber: The passing electron ionizes an atom; the atom acts as an impurity; a water droplet condenses around the impurity, forming a tiny but visible marker in the air. A series of these droplets form a vapor trail, marking the path of the electron.

Without an observer to consciously inspect that trail of droplets, no detection has taken place. All that has happened is that an electron has interacted with some atoms. Each one of those interactions has its own wave function of probability. Unobserved, each atom along the path of the electron is actually in a superposed ionized/unionized state. The moving electron has not experienced a collapse of its own wave function. Rather, its trajectory (which is only a wave function of probability, not a discrete state) has actually created a whole new series of wave functions. That is why a "detection" by an unconscious mechanism is not an observation at all; it merely creates an *endless regression* of uncollapsed wave functions. Only when a conscious observer looks into the cloud chamber does the entire system of electrons, atoms, and water droplets collapse to a discrete state.

As bizarre as it sounds, this view of reality is demanded by the Schrödinger wave function equation, which is confirmed by experimentation. Physicists don't know exactly when or how consciousness enters the detection process and collapses the wave function. But it is clear that consciousness is required in order for an observation to take place. A Geiger counter is not conscious, nor is a cloud chamber. To collapse the wave function of an electron—or a universe—you *must* have an intelligent observer (or Observer with a capital O). In order for reality to become real, *you must have a conscious SOUL as a witness.*

We have just glimpsed a profound insight into the meaning of the cosmos, into why it exists—and why *we* exist as immortal souls. The universe, it would seem, is made for souls by a Cosmic Soul. I submit that it is the observership of that Cosmic Soul that has made the universe real and discrete since long before the first human soul took shape upon the earth.

"*R*ight now, at this very moment (according to the MWI), there are literally millions of yous following millions of paths of reality that have branched at every decision-point in your life. There are paths of reality in which you are married to a different mate, in which you are pursuing a different career, in which you are poor, rich, obscure, famous, living it up, and dead as a doornail."

Here we sense a resonance of one of the fundamental truths of all the world's great theistic religions: Human souls are a miniature reflection of the soul of their maker. Through the act of conscious observation, human souls participate with the soul of the Cosmic Designer in actualizing the universe. The existence of the universe requires the existence of consciousness, and consciousness requires the existence of souls.

If this is your first excursion into the quantum realm, you may find this evidence for the soul more confusing than convincing. That's all right. The most convincing evidence of all is straight ahead.

A hard core of evidence

As we saw earlier, science fiction writer Isaac Asimov saw himself as nothing more than a temporary arrangement of molecules. In his 1978 book *Quasar, Quasar, Burning Bright*, he added:

As far as I know, there is not one piece of evidence ever advanced that would offer any hope that death is anything other than the permanent dissolution of the personality and that beyond it, as far as individual consciousness is concerned, there is nothing.

If you want to argue the point, present the evidence. I must warn you, though, that there are some arguments I won't accept.

I won't accept any argument from authority. ("The Bible says so.")

I won't accept any argument from internal conviction. ("I have faith it's so.")

I won't accept any argument from personal abuse. ("What are you, an atheist?")

I won't accept any argument from irrelevance. ("Do you think you have been put on this Earth just to exist for a moment of time?")

I won't accept any argument from anecdote. ("My cousin has a friend who went to a medium and talked to her dead husband.")

And when all that (and other varieties of non-evidence) are eliminated, there turns out to be nothing.

Then why do people believe? Because they want to.[7]

I've been an Asimov fan since I discovered his robot stories when I was no more than ten years old. I was saddened when the Good Doctor died in 1992. During his lifetime, he was not wrong about much, but I believe he was completely mistaken about the nonexistence of his own soul.

In a footnote to the passage quoted above, Asimov added, "Lately, there have been detailed reports about what people are supposed to have seen during 'clinical death.' I don't believe a word of it." I can empathize with his point of view. For years, I didn't think much of such reports myself. I had no intention of discussing "near-death experiences" (NDEs) when I began writing this book. It's not that I thought NDE survivors were lying about their experiences. But I was convinced that NDEs were entirely subjective experiences, not open to objective verification.

Sure, there were common elements among NDE reports that gave them a resonance of truth. Most reports included one or more of the following features: rising up and looking down on one's own body from somewhere near the ceiling; a sensation of rushing down a long tunnel and arriving in a place of brilliant light; a sense of peace and love; a life review; being greeted by deceased family members or by God; being told that "it's not your time yet" or "you still have work to do" and being sent back to the body.

But some NDE accounts sounded pretty flaky. For example, what are we to make of the woman who, after going into cardiac arrest during surgery, emerges from the tunnel and finds herself led into the light by....*Elvis*? In recent years, much of the media coverage of NDEs has been on the same level as Elvis sightings—sensational tales printed on the tabloid pages alongside alien abductions, two-headed babies, and the latest kinky doings of Hollywood celebs. But in my research for this book, I came across a hard core of case histories that I found impossible to rationalize away.

In these pages, I will present evidence that, in my opinion, clinches the case for the soul and for life after death. In accordance with Isaac Asimov's wishes, I won't argue from authority, internal conviction, personal abuse, or irrelevance. Any anecdotal evidence I present will not be of the "my cousin's friend went to a medium" variety. It is well-attested data gathered by scientifically trained observers—the kind of evidence even Isaac Asimov would accept. This evidence has made a believer out of me.

The soul at the point of death

NDE stories have been recorded for centuries, but it is only in recent decades, with the advance of lifesaving technology, that so many people have been able to set one foot over the threshold of death, then return to tell their stories. As recently as the mid-twentieth century, people who reported NDEs were hospitalized for mental disorders. But in 1976, with the publication of Raymond Moody's *Life After Life*, it became clear that near-death experiences are a real (though hard-to-quantify) phenomenon.

One of the most striking effects of NDEs is the transformed lives of NDEers. Call it an epiphany, a satori, a conversion—near-death survivors emerge forever changed by the experience. Those who once *believed* in God now say they *know*. Atheists are transformed into believers. Alcoholics and addicts shed their addictions. Materialists lose all interest in status and possessions. An NDE is a life-altering experience.

Another extraordinary feature of an NDE is that it appears so real that the NDEer is utterly convinced of its genuineness. Many call it the most vivid experience of their lives—so real that what we call "reality" seems dreamlike by comparison. Perhaps this is why so many NDEers lose interest in material things and pursuits. It may also explain why many NDEers report no feelings of fear while separated from their bodies. As M. Scott Peck observes, "Being immortal and pure spirit, the soul does not worry the least about the body, even the body's death."[8]

Dr. Michael Sabom reports the case of a construction worker from Georgia who needed emergency open-chest heart surgery without an anesthetic. Instead of describing terror and pain, the patient reported:

> That was the most beautiful instant in the whole world when I came out of that body!...I could see they [the doctors and nurses] were busy. In fact, one time a nurse I could see looked me right in the face just this far away [indicating one foot]. I tried to say something but she didn't say nothing....She was like looking at a movie screen that can't talk back and that doesn't recognize you're there. I was the real one and she was unreal. That's the way I felt.[9]

To this man, his out-of-body world was vividly real. Our own "real" world was unreal. That is an experience commonly reported by NDEers.

Do I consider these reports proof of the soul? No. Subjective experiences prove nothing. These stories *may* be actual peephole glimpses into the afterlife—but they are not scientific proof. At this point, we haven't crossed the evidence threshold Isaac Asimov set for us.

Some scientists suggest that NDEs could have a purely physiological origin. Neuroscientist Michael A. Persinger of Laurentian University in Sudbury, Ontario, has reproduced a number of NDE-like sensations (moving through a tunnel and seeing brilliant lights) by stimulating the brain's right temporal lobe with electromagnetic fields. Persinger concludes, "There's nothing magical about the NDE."[10] Other researchers have related other aspects of NDEs to natural opiates in the brain (endorphins), oxygen deprivation, fevers, seizures, medications, and so forth. In short, these researchers believe NDEs are mere hallucinations.

But NDEs are not so easily explained away. A substantial number of NDEs occur when a person has a completely flat electroencephalogram (EEG)—in short, when there is *no brain activity*. How could a person hallucinate in the absence of brain activity? Another problem is that careful researchers have interviewed patients who have experienced both hallucinations and NDEs, and these patients report that there is a clear difference between the two experiences.[11]

Astronomer Carl Sagan, in his book *Broca's Brain: Reflections on the Romance of Science*, suggested that NDEs may be nothing more than a recapitulation of the birth experience—an experience in which

> ...the child's head has penetrated the cervix and might, even if the eyes are closed, perceive a tunnel illuminated at one end and sense the brilliant radiance of the extrauterine world. The discovery of light for a creature that has lived its entire existence in darkness must be a profound and on some level an unforgettable experience. And there, dimly made out by the low resolution of the newborn's eyes, is some godlike figure surrounded by a halo of light—the Midwife or the Obstetrician or the Father. At the end of a monstrous travail, the baby flies away from the uterine universe, and rises toward the lights and the gods.[12]

A few moments' consideration, however, quickly dashes Sagan's theory: It is not the baby's face but the crown of the head that faces the birth canal. A faded memory of the birth process could hardly account for the intensely vivid impressions described by NDEers.

And there is even worse news for skeptics: An important number of NDE cases actually go beyond the subjective anecdote, providing *objective verification* of a soul that exists apart from the body.

Soul survivors

Kimberly Clark Sharp was in her early twenties when she died—and lived to tell about it.

On May 25, 1970, she went to the Department of Motor Vehicles in Shawnee Mission, Kansas, to apply for a driver's license. While waiting in line with her father, she became dizzy and pale. On her way out of the DMV building, Kimberly collapsed on the sidewalk in front of the entrance, blocking the doors. A uniformed nurse happened to be nearby and rushed over to help. Kneeling at Kimberly's side, the nurse became alarmed when she could detect no pulse and no breathing. Kimberly appeared dead.

Within minutes, fire department paramedics arrived. They brought with them a brand-new portable ventilator—so new, in fact, that it was still in the packaging. They broke open the packaging and removed the machine—then there was a brief argument about how it should be used. The ventilator had two settings—one to ventilate (force air into the patient's lungs), and the other to aspirate (suck liquid or obstructions out of a blocked airway). Being unfamiliar with the machine, the paramedics operated it incorrectly, aspirating instead of ventilating, causing Kimberly's lungs to collapse.

The paramedics tried to revive her, but after several minutes with no vital signs, they turned to Kimberly's distraught father and said, "There's nothing more we can do." Just then, a man pushed through the gathering crowd of onlookers, shoving the paramedics aside. He immediately began mouth-to-mouth resuscitation. After a few minutes of this, the man swore and said, "I'm not getting a thing!" But he continued to work on her, pounding her chest and willing his breath into her lungs.

And she began to breathe. A cheer went up from the crowd. As soon as Kimberly was stable enough to transport, the paramedics put her into an ambulance. Her father climbed in, and they took off for the hospital. She later pieced the story together from what her father and her doctors told her.

"After they got me to the emergency room," she told me in a recent phone interview, "things continued to go wrong, and it was very iffy for a while. The total resuscitation effort, both the time I was on the sidewalk and the time I spent in the emergency room, took about an hour and a half. So I had quite a prolonged NDE."

I asked Kimberly what she saw and felt while she was dead. She described an acute sense of awareness of her surroundings. For example, she was aware of the nurse who knelt to help her. "The first thing I remember after I collapsed," she told me, "was that a woman was kneeling on my left. She was saying, 'I'm not getting a pulse!' I couldn't see her, but I could hear her very clearly. So I said to her, 'Of course you're getting a pulse, or I wouldn't be talking to you.' But she couldn't hear me. She just kept saying that I had no pulse, no respiration. And when the paramedics arrived, they said the same thing.

"I became amused and a bit flustered about this. I wondered, *How can they be talking about me like this? I'm talking and they can't hear me, and they keep saying I'm not breathing! But I've never felt better in my life!* At that moment, I had a sense of well-being I never knew existed. I felt great. Finally, I decided to stop trying to persuade everybody I was alive. They were ignoring me anyway, so I just decided to let go. As soon as I made that decision, I felt myself in a completely different environment—a warm, comfortable, *safe* place. I know there are emotions in that place, because I felt a sense of relief.

"Although I couldn't see anyone, I knew I wasn't alone. I was surrounded by a dense foggy substance. I had a sense that I was waiting for something—not with anxiety, but with a calm, secure sense of anticipation. Earthly time had no meaning—there was no 'before' or 'after.' Past, present, and future seemed to exist simultaneously.

"By adjusting my vision, I could see something through the foggy masses—I could see brilliant lights, black holes, holes with depth like bottomless pits. With a shift or adjustment of my vision, the gray fog around me became something that was not a formless fog but a vast blending of dark particles and penetrating light. I *knew* I was in a place that really existed—it was not dreamlike or unreal.

"In the midst of this came the Light.

"Words cannot do justice to the Light I experienced. It just exploded underneath me with incredible power and energy, brighter than a hundred suns, yet I wasn't afraid of it. It was like standing on the Earth while it detonated, yet I was unharmed. It was an immense power, brighter than our sun. I could see in every direction, and the Light was expanding endlessly and doubling back on itself. I knew I was perceiving eternity, not just linear eternity but dimensional eternity. And I knew that the Light was made up entirely of love. If I had been in the presence of that Light in my physical body, I would have been dissolved—I could not have withstood it.

"I also knew I was in the presence of what we call God. I think there's a lot of wisdom in the Jewish tradition which says that the name of God cannot be spoken. It is impossible to grasp God with words. I communicated with the light, but it was not a conversation in English.

The only way I can describe it is that it was a conversation in mathematics and music."

I asked Kimberly approximately how long this conversation went on. There was laughter in her reply. "Approximately forever," she said. "It was endless. I was told things that had never entered my consciousness before. I asked question after question: What is life? What is the point of our existence? Why are we here? And I received answer after answer: We are here to learn to love others. Our soul demands it. Our soul must learn—that's its job. Our earthly existence is a good place in which to learn; it's a school from which everyone graduates.

"I asked why we had to die. If God could laugh—Well, God *does* laugh! God's amused answer to my question was that we came from somewhere and we are going somewhere. Meanwhile, what matters is now. Life is important and valuable, a sacred gift, not to be taken lightly.

"I asked why there's so much pain and suffering. The answer: Suffering is a fast track to God. It's terrible, but true. Our soul learns best under duress. When do we pray? Not when we are on a beach in Hawaii, having our backs rubbed with coconut oil, but when we are wracked with physical, emotional, or spiritual pain.

"Then God told me the worst thing possible: I was being sent back! I said 'No! I don't want to go back!' Now, it's okay to argue with God, of course. God will always win, but it's okay. When my argument with God was over, I was sent back—but I missed my body.

"The thing is, I have a problem with spatial skills. For example, I flunked parallel parking because I couldn't get within four feet of the curb. The same thing happened when I was sent back to my body—I missed it by four feet! I had just had the most sacred experience of my existence, and when I came back, I couldn't even park *myself*!"

From outside her own body, Kimberly could see the man working on her, giving her mouth-to-mouth resuscitation after the paramedics had given up. As she took her first breath on her own, she rejoined her body. She actually passed through the man as she did so. As she went through him, she sensed his compassion toward her.

From the moment she reentered her body until her arrival at the hospital, she remembers almost nothing—but what happened next is sharply etched in her memory. "Once I got to the hospital," she told me, "things weren't going well for me. I was comatose—but I felt fully conscious and trapped in my body. It was corpse-cold, like something out of the House of Usher. It was dark, dank, creepy, endless—a real night-mare."

As she lay in this state, she felt God come to her in her darkness. This time there was no explosion of light—just a quiet communication. "I felt God saying, 'All right, if you really want to die, fine. You have free will, it's your choice.' Not in words, of course, but that was the sense of it. Then a window opened to my right, and through that window I saw an endless panorama, a blue-green sea of grass under an intensely blue sky. The colors were rich and saturated, like Crayola colors. It was balmy and warm, and I knew that each of those blades of grass had consciousness and awareness.

"I realized that the window was my border. I could go through it—but if I did, I wouldn't come back. I thought, *Okay, I'm going*. And God said, 'Before you do that, look.' And in a series of flashes, I saw my future—if I chose to live it. I saw a place where the mountain meets the water; I now know it was a glimpse of Seattle, where I now live. I saw myself engaged in acts of helping others. And I thought, *That looks like an interesting future*. I had always been shallow and materialistic—not the kind of person who devotes herself to serving others. But the future I was shown was so attractive, I chose to live."

After her recovery, Kimberly earned a master's degree in social work and became a critical care social worker. She didn't know how to catego-rize what she had been through. She had never heard of NDEs—in fact, the term "near-death experience" did not yet exist. She felt she existed partly *inside* her body, and partly *beyond* her body. On that basis, she decided that she must be a "high-functioning schizophrenic."

Then, in April 1977, something happened that completely changed her world. "I was a social worker in the critical care unit at Harborview Medical Center, a very large and busy Level One trauma center that serves Alaska, Washington, Idaho, and Montana. While I was working there, I met Maria, a Spanish-speaking migrant worker from the Yakima Valley area. She had come to Seattle on a visit and suffered a heart attack her first day in the city.

"Maria became my patient after she was admitted to the coronary care unit. It was my job to get her an interpreter, contact her family, get her some personal items she would need, and so forth. Between her pid-gin English and my pidgin Spanish, we managed to communicate rea-sonably well. Three days after she arrived in my unit, Maria went into cardiac arrest. Harborview is a teaching hospital, so the piercing sound from the heart monitor brought a dozen people running—thirteen, counting myself. Maria was full flatline, and it was scary for a few minutes, but the resuscitation was fairly easy. Finally, they had her breathing on her own, though she was unconscious. There wasn't anything more for me to do, so I left.

"At the end of my workday, I was called into Maria's room. She was very agitated, which is dangerous for a coronary patient. My job was to figure out what she needed so she could rest. She pointed to a corner of the ceiling and told me she had floated there and watched the doctors working on her when she was in cardiac arrest. She named the doctors who had worked on her. She described the equipment in the room at the time, such as the EKG machine. She mentioned that people kept kicking the paper that scrolled from the EKG machine. And she was right on all counts.

"I didn't want to believe Maria, because I had never really accepted my own NDE as a valid experience. I was sure Maria's story had a 'rational explanation.' How did she know which doctors were in the room while she was unconscious? Well, hearing is the last thing to go, so maybe she recognized their voices. How did she know about the EKG paper on the floor? Just a lucky guess. I did Maria a great disservice, trying to dismiss her story. I had mentally stuffed my own NDE, and Maria's story was too close to my own—and too threatening. I had never met anyone else with a story like mine, and I thought I was crazy. I had once seen a woman taken to a psychiatric lockup after she described an out-of-body experience, and that horrified me—it still does. So I wanted to disprove Maria's story.

"She told me that while she was in an out-of-body state, she could 'think' herself to another place—and *boom*, she would be there. She went outside her window and floated there, then she hovered above the emergency room entrance. Then she 'thought' herself over to a different part of the hospital, where she came eyeball to shoelace with a blue tennis shoe. It was perched on a ledge, about three or four stories above the ground. She said the little-toe part of the shoe was scuffed, and the lace was tucked under the sole. She was agitated because she wanted someone to find the shoe and confirm that she wasn't crazy. As fate would have it, that someone was me.

"I went outside and looked up at the wall of the west side of the building, where Maria said she had seen the shoe. I didn't see anything—but if it was on a ledge, it might not be visible from the ground. So I went inside and went from room to room, looking through windows. I had to press my head up against the window in order to look down at the ledge. After checking several windows, I caught sight of something I fully expected *not* to see. It was a man's tennis shoe, navy blue, sitting on the ledge.

"I thought I was losing my last grasp of sanity. Everything went into slow-mo. I got very calm, and I remember thinking, *I can explain this.* Looking out the window, I could see a lone downtown building a half mile away. I thought, *Maybe Maria went up in that building, looked through a telescope in this direction, saw a blue tennis shoe on the ledge, could even see the scuff on the toe, and she remembered every detail just in case she got a massive heart attack, and had to come to Harborview Medical Center. Sure, that makes perfect sense!* I was grasping for any rational explanation.

"Then my mouth opened and words flew out: 'This happened to me!' I didn't even realize what I was saying until I had said it. Instantly, I lost my sense of being able to stand, and I fell against the glass—I remember my breath fogging the window momentarily. Then I recovered my composure, opened the window, and retrieved the shoe. I examined it closely. It was exactly as Maria had described it. And it was clear that the only way she could have seen the scuffed toe and the shoestring tucked under the sole was if she had been floating right outside and at very close range to the shoe. I had exhausted all my rationalizations. It had to be true.

"I took the shoe back to Maria's room and showed it to her. Her face lit up with the joy of recognition. That shoe became a little shrine at Harborview Medical Center, like Seattle's own Shroud of Turin. It was a highly witnessed event, and there are still people at Harborview today who were there when Maria flatlined, and who saw the shoe."

This incident is representative of a small but important class of NDEs that provide objective verification of a subjective experience. The *only* kind of NDE that can objectively verify the existence of the soul is the kind in which the NDEer gains knowledge that could not have been acquired *except* by an out-of-body experience. A number of such incidences have been documented by various observers, including Kimberly herself.

Since that 1977 incident, Kimberly has conducted face-to-face interviews with over two thousand NDE survivors. She describes many of those cases, as well as her own story and the story of Maria, in her book *After the Light: The Spiritual Path to Purpose* (Morrow 1995). In 1982, Kimberly founded the Seattle chapter of the International Association for Near-Death Studies (website at http://www.seattleiands.org/). Many of the stories Kimberly has uncovered are stories like Maria's—stories with objectively verifiable details that prove that NDEs are much more than mere subjective experiences and hallucinations.

The most rational explanation

No one has made a more intensive study of the dying process than Elisabeth Kübler-Ross. Her specialty was in comforting critically injured children and talking to them as they approached death. She was impressed that these children were invariably aware of other family members who preceded them in death. Kübler-Ross would sit with the dying child, watch silently and hold the child's hand. In many cases, she observed that a child in obvious pain would experience "a peaceful serenity, which is always an ominous sign." In *On Children and Death*, she writes,

> Shortly before children die there is often a very "clear moment," as I call it. Those who have remained in a coma since the accident or after surgery open their eyes and seem very coherent. Those who have had great pain and discomfort are very quiet and at peace. It is in those moments that I asked them if they were willing to share with me what they were experiencing.[13]

She recounts one such case, in which a family was involved in a terrible car wreck. The mother was killed at the scene, and her two sons were rushed to different hospitals. Sitting at the bedside of the younger boy, Kübler-Ross saw him awaken from a coma. The ominous "clear moment" had arrived. The child, though in pain, was quiet and at peace. Kübler-Ross asked the boy how he felt. His response, as she relates in her book:

> "Yes, everything is all right now. Mommy and Peter are already waiting for me," [the boy] replied. With a content little smile, he slipped back into a coma from which he made the transition we call death.

I was quite aware that his mother had died at the scene of the accident, but Peter had not died. He had been brought to a special burn unit in another hospital severely burnt, because the car had caught fire before he was extricated from the wreck. Since I was only collecting data, I accepted the boy's information and determined to look in on Peter. It was not necessary, however, because as I passed the nursing station there was a call from the other hospital to inform me that Peter had died a few minutes earlier.[14]

The boy could not have possibly known that his brother Peter was dead—yet he *did* know. What's more, this was not an isolated case. Kübler-Ross had seen it happen many times before. In fact, in all her years of sitting at the bedsides of dying children, she said she had observed that

...every single child who mentioned that someone was waiting for them mentioned a person who had actually preceded them in death, even if by only a few moments. And yet none of these children had been informed of the recent death of the relatives by us at any time. Coincidence? By now there is no scientist or statistician who could convince me that this occurs, as some colleagues claim, as "a result of oxygen deprivation" or for other "rational and scientific" reasons.[15]

That is an astounding observation, made by a highly respected clinician who understands the process of dying as well as anyone who has ever lived.

Born in Switzerland in 1926, Elisabeth Kübler-Ross first confronted the horrors of wholesale death as a volunteer relief worker at Maidenek, a Nazi death camp, immediately after the end of World War II. There she saw boxcars filled with little shoes taken from murdered Jewish children. Inside the grim wooden barracks of Maidenek, she saw the most poignant and heartbreaking sight of all: pictures of butterflies scratched into the rough wood by the doomed children. The butterflies symbolized freedom and rebirth. The image of the butterfly became a central symbol in her life.

At the end of *On Children and Death*, she says that her goal in life is to let people know—not merely believe, but *know*—"that our physical body is truly only the cocoon, the outer shell of the human being. Our inner, true self, the 'butterfly,' is immortal and indestructible and is freed at the moment we call death."[16]

And that is what I want you to be assured of as well. I know the soul is real because my friend Kim Alexis received the gift of a farewell visit from a friend on his way to eternity. I know the soul is real because the universe needs souls in order to become real and discrete. I know the soul is real because only a living soul could know the things that so many near-death survivors have known. Most of all, I know that at the threshold of death, what we now call "reality" suddenly becomes unreal—and what now seems unreal to us suddenly becomes reality. The evidence is overwhelming.

To those few who, despite the evidence, insist that there must be "a rational explanation," I say, of course there is. The soul is *real*—and that's the most rational explanation of all.

18

Does Prayer Really Work?

Fred Judkins and I have a lot in common.

Fred was my roommate in college. We're exactly the same age, both born on May 9, 1953. We both love movies, especially old monster movies and Marx Brothers comedies. We have similar philosophies of life. Even our contrasts made us compatible as roommates. Since our tastes in music were so different, I could never blame him for scratches on my vinyl disks of The Who and The Doors, and he could never accuse me of wearing out his Gilbert and Sullivan collection. I have always marveled at Fred's quick comedic mind—a nimble, high-octane, turbocharged wit that invariably left my poor plodding intellect in the dust.

After college, Fred followed his love for movies all the way to Hollywood (well, technically Burbank). Over the years, he has worked as a sound editor for a number of studios, including Disney and Twentieth Century-Fox, and we've always kept in touch. In fact, our family once got to watch him at work in the Hitchcock Theater at Universal Studios, creating sound effects for the comedy-thriller *Mystery Men*.

I can't describe the shock and devastation I felt in September 1998 when I heard that Fred was in the hospital, battling for his life against leukemia. I later talked to Fred about that terrible time—and about the prayers that got him through it.

"They don't call it 'nuclear medicine' for nothing"

"My symptoms began in July 1998," he told me. "My gums were swelling, and my dentist said I had a bacterial infection. The symptoms became acute in August. My gums were worse, and I had lymph node swelling in my neck. If I'd had a blood test in July, I would have been diagnosed right away. For some reason, the doctors didn't do that until September. I came home one night and found phone messages from two medical labs, telling me my white count was off the charts. The doctor wanted to put me in the hospital right away for a week of tests. I said no. I needed that week to get my affairs in order—just in case."

I asked Fred what was going through his mind at the time.

"I had a lot of fear about specific medical procedures," he said. "I had rarely been sick before, so this was new and scary. The first bad day was when they went in to chip out a piece of my tailbone. It was all I could do to keep from running into the street. I told myself, 'Don't look at what they are doing to you. Just pray to get through it.' So I prayed, 'God, I can't endure this, but please give me the strength to endure it anyway.' I couldn't whip up any faith or strength on my own, but I had a strong sense that God was superintending everything."

As Fred started treatment, his wife used the Internet to contact relatives and friends. "Immediately, my name was on prayer lists at our church and other churches," he recalled. "Requests came in from friends wanting e-mail updates. I found out there is a network of people all over the world who do nothing but pray for cancer patients. Suddenly, this huge cushion of prayer ballooned all around me—it was really remarkable.

"Most of the people praying for me were Christians, but a Jewish coworker was also praying for me. So was my Mormon neighbor. And another friend of mine who is into Eastern religion was offering prayers for me. People just rallied around me—people from the film industry, people I used to work with and hadn't seen in years. There was a blood drive at Disney, and the Disney post-production department had an original Disney painting done, showing Mickey Mouse and me running down the corridor together—that really lifted my spirits. It was all so amazing and humbling.

"The doctors didn't expect me to survive 'induction,' the first wave of chemotherapy. They install a tube in your chest so they can put everything right into the tubing. Then they give you as much chemo as they can without killing you. My hematologist called the procedure 'going to hell and coming back.' It kills off the cancer cells, then your bone marrow has to regenerate itself. A lot of people don't survive induction. They don't call it 'nuclear medicine' for nothing. The doctor said, 'We're going to give you the same thing they gave Sadaam Hussein'—and I thought he was kidding!

"My immune system had crashed by the time I was diagnosed, so I had developed a near-fatal lung infection called aspergillis. When I started treatment, my internal organs were in such bad shape that I couldn't make it up a flight of stairs. After I began induction, the chemo started killing off my internal organs, and I dropped fifty pounds right away. After the induction, they removed my gall bladder and did a lung biopsy—then came the second wave of chemo. The first wave kills off the leukemia, but it comes back quickly, so they give you a second round and a third.

"The side effects from the chemo were terrible, but not as bad as many people get. I had nerve damage, shingles, numbness, incontinence, muscle atrophy, weight loss, and short-term memory loss. I couldn't re-member what I did for a living, or even how to turn on a computer. The biggest blessing is that the nausea problem isn't as bad as it once was—they can just put you out. The worst thing about cancer is that you get to watch yourself die slowly—it's pretty grim.

"But during that first wave of induction, when I was really sick, I had this amazing sense of God's presence. When you go through some-thing like that, you know when God is near. As sick as I was, I knew the difference between being close to God and being high on painkillers. This was really like being *in* heaven but not able to *see* heaven. It's a gift. It's an assurance that God is walking through your life with you. And it's an awareness that people around the world are alongside you, praying for you.

"It's been a wild ride—but the wildest thing of all is knowing that the great Lord of Creation is interested in the details of our lives. Yes, it was a horrible thing to go through. Yes, I'm still scared of needles and drills and the things they stuck down my throat. But I've had God walk through my life with me. His closeness in that time was like a preview of coming attractions."

Fred believes it was prayer that brought him through the horrors of cancer and chemotherapy—but is there any *objective* data to support what Fred *subjectively* believes to be true? Can it be *proven* that prayer works? Stories about seemingly answered prayer are interesting but ultimately unpersuasive. But what if there were evidence—strong, convincing, *sci-entific* evidence—that prayer really does work? What if Fred's subjective experience of answered prayer could be objectively corroborated?

The science of prayer

When I was about fifteen, my Uncle Chet was seriously ill with cancer. Except for the death of my grandfather when I was two, I had never lost a loved one before. I hardly ever thought about death. I knew next to nothing about cancer. When my Uncle Chet became ill, I could tell from my mother's concern that the situation was serious. But our entire family was praying for Uncle Chet, and I knew that everything was going to turn out all right. I remember a conversation I had with my cousin Cliff (also one of Chet's nephews) about the situation. Cliff and I talked it over, and decided that, with so many people praying, Chet was sure to recover.

It was only a few weeks later that Chet passed away at the age of fifty-four. I was stunned and bewildered. How was that possible? We had prayed so faithfully! How could God say no to all of our prayers? How could God let such a terrible thing happen to such a good man? I'll never forget what a blow that was to my young faith. Ever since that first disappointment with God, I have been seeking answers to this deep mystery called prayer. I'm happy to report that I have found some of the answers I sought.

Almost any medical researcher will tell you that prayer has the power to heal people—about the same power as a sugar pill. That kind of healing power is called "the placebo effect," the mysterious power to fool the mind into helping the body heal itself. If you believe that the little pink pill you are taking is a powerful new wonder drug, then you will probably get better, even if the pill is nothing but sugar. In the same way, if you believe prayer works, then prayer will probably speed your recovery from an illness or injury, even if prayer is nothing but words mumbled into the great unfeeling emptiness of the universe. So goes the usual scientific reasoning.

Prayer is also known to be beneficial to the body through stress-reduction and relaxation. Doctors report that patients who pray and meditate experience lower blood pressure, fewer gastrointestinal problems, improved pain management ability, and other health benefits. But placebo effects and stress-reduction techniques are hardly miraculous, and such benefits do not have anything to do with whether or not God really answers prayer. The big question is: Does prayer truly call forth the active, dynamic involvement of God in human lives?

"Unequivocally, yes," says Dr. Larry Dossey, an internist and author of *Healing Words: The Power of Prayer and The Practice of Medicine* (HarperCollins, 1993). "I base this answer not just on faith, but on the outcome of scores of scientific studies."

The most carefully documented of those studies was published by cardiologist Randolph Byrd in the *Southern Medical Journal* in 1988. Over a ten-month period from August 1982 through May 1983, Dr. Byrd randomly chose (using a computer-generated list) 393 patients from the coronary care unit at San Francisco General Hospital. These patients were divided into two groups. One group was prayed for by home prayer groups; the second group was not prayed for. Prayer was directed to the Judeo-Christian God by prayer volunteers from both Protestant and Roman Catholic churches. Each patient in the prayed-for group had from three to seven prayer volunteers, who were given the patient's first name and diagnosis. Each prayer volunteer was asked to pray daily and specifically for a speedy recovery and for the prevention of complications.

> *"The big question is: Does prayer truly call forth the active, dynamic involvement of God in human lives?"*

It was a carefully constructed "double-blind" experiment: Neither the patients nor their physicians and nurses knew which group the patients were in—prayed-for or not-prayed-for. The results were startling. The study found that the prayed-for patients were five times less likely to require antibiotics than the not-prayed-for group; they were three times less likely to develop pulmonary edema (fluid in the lungs). Prayed-for patients also "had fewer episodes of pneumonia, had fewer cardiac arrests, and were less frequently intubated and ventilated."[1]

A process called "multivariate analysis" was used to group all the variables of the study into meaningful patterns of statistical relationships. This analysis helps determine how statistically significant the findings are. (The standard level of statistical significance in scientific studies is recognized as one chance in 500—statisticians refer to this as a "p value of less than 0.05" or $p < 0.05$). If the multivariate analysis yielded a low statistical significance, it would mean that the test results were not much different than you would expect from random chance. But multivariate analysis of the Byrd study showed something extraordinary.

The Byrd study showed a statistical significance of *one chance in 10,000* (or $p < 0.0001$). In short, the findings were so significant, the differences between the not-prayed-for and prayed-for groups were so dramatic, that the odds of those findings occurring by sheer random chance are *one in 10,000*. Very few scientific studies ever reach such a high level of statistical significance.

Nearly every parameter measured by Dr. Byrd's study was shown to be affected by prayer. Additionally, Dr. Byrd noted that there was no way to know how many people in the "not-prayed-for" group were actually being prayed for by friends or relatives who were not part of the study. If it were possible to completely isolate the "not-prayed-for" group from all possibility of being prayed for, the results might have been even more dramatic.

Eleven years later, *The Archives of Internal Medicine* published another study on the effects of intercessory prayer on coronary care patients.[2] This controlled trial, conducted by Dr. William H. Harris (a Ph.D. heart-disease researcher) and eight colleagues at Saint Luke's Hospital in Kansas City, Missouri, was even larger than the San Francisco General study. It involved 990 patients with life-threatening heart conditions (from heart attacks to coronary heart disease to congestive heart failure). Of these patients, 466 were randomly assigned to the IP (intercessory prayer) group, while 524 were randomly assigned to a control (no prayer) group.

This Kansas City trial was even more "blind" than the San Francisco General study. Doctors and patients in the San Francisco study knew that a clinical trial was being conducted, but did not know which individuals were assigned to which group. But doctors and patients in the Kansas City study *were not even told* that a study was being conducted, eliminating all possibility of bias. Seventy-five people were chosen from various Protestant and Catholic churches to pray for the patients in the IP group, and the prayers were conducted remotely, not at the hospital. The intercessors (the people who prayed) were only told (1) the patient's first name and (2) that the person was ill. No details of the illness were disclosed. The intercessors were instructed to pray for each patient for twenty-eight days.

The patients of both the IP group and the control group were evaluated according to thirty-five medical measurements, from the types of medications they required to length of hospitalization to speed of recovery to outcome (survival or death). Results: The IP group scored 11 percent better than the control group patients—a result that is considered statistically significant. "This is a very well-designed study and it is very well-written," said James Dalen, dean of the Arizona University School of Medicine and editor of *The Archives of Internal Medicine*. "If this was a medication, the conclusion would be that this medication helped."[3]

The Kansas City study confirmed the results of Dr. Randolph Byrd's study at San Francisco General. These two clinical trials are the only double-blind, peer-reviewed studies conducted on the healing power of prayer. The results of both trials are clear and persuasive: Prayer really does work.

The next obvious question is *how* does prayer work? What is the *mechanism* behind the power of prayer? Neither of these studies attempted to answer the question. "This trial," concludes Dr. Harris, "was designed to explore not a mechanism but a phenomenon....We have not proven that God answers prayer or that God even exists. It was intercessory prayer, not the existence of God, that was tested here. All we have observed is that when individuals outside of the hospital speak (or think) the first names of hospitalized patients with an attitude of prayer, the latter appeared to have a 'better' CCU experience."[4]

I want to underscore the fact that *patients should not abandon medical treatment in favor of prayer alone.* These studies show that prayer works in concert with the best available medical treatment—*not* in place of medical treatment. Prayer is certainly not a substitute for bypass surgery or chemotherapy or an emergency appendectomy.

Another thing to keep in mind: Prayer does not guarantee any particular outcome. Even though friends and family are praying for them and even though they pray for themselves, well people do get sick, sick people do get even sicker, and eventually everyone dies. Prayer is not a form of magic, and it does not place the total outcome within human control. All we know for sure is that prayer can influence the outcome in many cases.

Closer than we suspect

When I met with Reggie White at his Knoxville home in 1996, one of the things we talked about is prayer. Reggie related that he first learned about the reality of prayer when he was a boy. "I was about ten years old," he told me, "and I thought God didn't answer kids' prayers, only adults' prayers. No one taught me that—I just figured in my own mind that God was too busy to pay attention to the prayers of children.

"I was playing in a youth baseball league, and we were up against a team with a real good pitcher. That kid could really zip the ball, and I could never get a hit off him. I was real intimidated by him. I came up to bat late in the game with two, maybe three guys on base. I remember the pitcher intentionally walking the batter ahead of me, saying I was going to be an easy out. We were behind, but we had a chance to win if I could knock in a run or two. So I stood in the batter's box and prayed, 'God, if you answer children's prayers, then please let me hit a home run.' I raised my bat and that kid pitched two strikes right over the plate. I thought, *Well, I guess I was right—God only answers prayers for grownups.*

"So the kid zipped another pitch, and I swung at it and connected. I was so shocked, because that ball was *gone*! I took off running and sprinted around the bases as fast as I could. I was hoping I could get a double, maybe a triple. Then I heard my coach yelling, 'Slow down, Reggie! You hit a home run!' After I crossed the plate, I thought, *Oh, man! God really does answer children's prayers!*

"The kids from the other team came up to me after the game. They said that when the ball hit the ground, it made a big hole. I thought, *Well, that must have been God!* That's when I really believed for the first time that God was real, and that he cared about me.

"Why did God give me that home run? Did he like me more than he liked the pitcher? No, God had something to teach me about himself, that's all. Maybe he had another lesson for the pitcher. But God wanted me to know that he is real and that he answers prayer—even for kids."

I learned a similar lesson when I was about eight years old. We lived in a small town in central California. I had to ride my bike three or four blocks to school. We lived near the edge of town and there was only one road to school. Along the way was a house with a pair of vicious dogs.

Every morning of my first week in the third grade, I rode past that house and those dogs would come tearing after me. They both had that deep-in-the-throat snarl that said they preferred human flesh over Purina Dog Chow. Each morning, I arrived at school sweating and terrified, heart pounding like a jackhammer.

At first, I didn't want my parents to know how scared I was. But after a few days, I told my dad about the dogs. "Tell you what, son," he said, "let's pray about this." So we prayed that the dogs would leave me alone.

The next morning, I got on my bike and rode off to school. I warily passed the house where the dogs lived, pedaling quickly to build up momentum before the chase began—but the dogs never appeared. Fact is, I was never troubled by those dogs again.

For years, whenever I doubted the reality of God, I often remembered how my prayer had been so convincingly answered when I was just eight years old. It wasn't until I was an adult that I remembered that incident—and got suspicious. I went to my dad and said, "Remember those two dogs that used to chase me on the way to school? We prayed for them to leave me alone, and they did."

"Yes," he said. "I remember."

"Did *you* have anything to do with that prayer being answered?"

He just smiled and changed the subject.

Now, some people might say, "God didn't answer your prayer. Your dad did." Fair enough. But I ask you: If a prayer can be answered through natural or human means, why shouldn't God do so? God may answer our prayers more often than we know—and the reason we don't realize it is that the answer to our prayers is sometimes closer than we suspect.

There is a story (stop me if you've heard it) about a man who was trapped in his house by a flood. As the waters rose, he prayed that God would save his life. Soon, a rescue worker came by in a boat and called out, "Get in the boat!" But the man said, "No, I have faith in God! He will save me!" So the rescue worker shrugged and rowed off to help someone else. The flood waters continued rising, and the man moved to the second floor. Another boat came by and the rescue worker called, "Get in the boat!" Again, the man refused. "God will save me!" The waters rose higher and the man climbed onto his roof. A helicopter came and dropped a rope, but the man refused to grab it. "God will save me!" he said. So the chopper flew off.

Soon, the flood waters engulfed the house and the man drowned. Arriving in heaven, the man confronted God and said, "I prayed to you! I trusted in you! Why didn't you save me?"

God shrugged. "What do you want from me? I sent you two boats and a helicopter."

When God answers your prayer, make sure you are open and receptive to whatever form that answer may take. And no matter when and how the answer comes, be grateful and amazed that the God of the universe takes a personal interest in *you*.

19

Do Miracles Really Happen?

I have a friend who has walked on fire.

He's a corporate CEO, and he and I were in his home near San Francisco a few years ago, working on a book together. As we talked, I happened to mention the name of motivational guru Tony Robbins. And he said, "Yeah, I know Tony. I fire-walked at one of his seminars."

My eyes widened to twice-normal-size. "You fire-walked?"

"Sure." He shrugged. "It was no big deal."

"No big deal! Is there some kind of trick to it?"

"No trick," he said. "The coals are hot, just like the coals in a barbecue pit. But anybody can fire-walk."

I asked him to explain.

"I went to one of Tony's 'Unleash the Power Within' seminars," he said. "Tony had his assistants stoke up a big wood fire. As it burned down to coals, they raked the coals into a fire-walking bed. Tony went into this big rah-rah 'mind revolution' talk. Now, I believe in positive thinking and motivation, but this was like a revival meeting.

"Tony shouted, 'How many of you came here to walk on fire?' and every hand went up. He got everyone clapping and chanting and all psyched up. Then, when things reached a fever pitch, he sent them, one by one, barefoot, across the bed of fire. He'd say, 'Don't look down! You're walking on a bed of cool moss!' People would walk the coals, and get a lot of applause and high-fives.

"I watched with a kind of clinical detachment, and I said to myself, 'There's nothing magical to this. There's a rational, scientific explanation. I don't know what it is, but I know it has nothing to do with mind power.' I decided if I just walked slowly and deliberately, I could fire-walk like everyone else."

So my friend walked the coals, and didn't get a burn or even a blister. How did he do it?

"To this day," he said, "I don't know how it works. Maybe it has to do with the sweat on the soles of your feet. Maybe there's some other explanation. But whatever it is, it's not magic."

Fire-walking has long been considered a miracle of faith. For example, every June 24, villagers of San Pedro Manrique, Spain, observe the Fiesta of San Juan with a centuries-old midnight fire-walking ceremony. Villagers fire-walk to show their faith in the Blessed Virgin. Fire-walkers often carry wives, mothers, or children on their backs as they walk the coals. Though they claim that the Blessed Virgin makes them invulnerable, they all use the same technique urged by Tony Robbins: Walk slowly and steadily, eyes straight ahead.

In case you're thinking of strolling barefoot through the backyard barbecue—*don't!* Some fire-walkers have gotten badly burned. For example, an insurance company held a motivational fire-walk at the Moathouse Hotel in Shurdington, England. As colleagues cheered, ten trainees walked through the fire and seven of the ten—six men and one woman—were burned badly enough to require hospitalization.[1]

Fire-walking looks like a miracle—but is it? Are fire-walkers protected by the power of faith? No. It's a simple matter of physics. David Willey, a physics professor at the University of Pittsburgh, has fire-walked numerous times and has only gotten one dime-sized blister. During one demonstration, he walked a 165-foot-long bed of coals three times without stopping—that's over one and one-half times the length of a football field!

"You wait until the fire is in the right state to do it," he explained on National Public Radio. "It's a matter of the wood's low thermal conductivity. Wood is a good insulator. Also, your feet don't conduct heat very well. So if you pick the right time, you can do it. If you pick the wrong time, you can burn quite seriously."[2]

The point is this: We human beings are easily conned into seeing miracles where no miracles exist. So, as we consider the question, "Do miracles really happen?" we need to maintain a healthy skepticism.

Irrational violation—or meaningful intervention?

The Scottish rationalist philosopher David Hume (1711–1776) defined *miracle* this way: "A miracle is a violation of the laws of nature."[3]

Hume's thinking continues to assert an enormous influence over scientific and philosophical thought in the twenty-first century. Most of today's rationalists find the idea of miracles not only laughable, but offensive. Why? Because, as Hume defines it, a miracle is a violation against reason, a rape of the laws of nature. Horror writer Stephen King put it this way:

> Go to your church and listen to your stories about Jesus walking on the water, but if I saw a guy doing that I'd scream and scream and scream. Because it wouldn't look like a miracle to me. It would look like an *offense*.[4]

If we accept Hume's definition of a miracle as a *violation* of the laws of nature, then I, too, would see miracles as an offense. My God-given intelligence revolts against the idea that the Cosmic Designer would make an orderly, rational universe, then disfigure its orderliness with irrational violations. In his book *Miracles*, C. S. Lewis states the objection this way:

> [God] might work miracles. But would He? Many people of sincere piety feel that He would not. They think it unworthy of Him. It is petty and capricious tyrants who break their own laws; good and wise kings obey them. Only an incompetent workman will produce work which needs to be interfered with.[5]

The scientific evidence shows us a Cosmic Designer who is clearly neither petty nor irrational. As Einstein said, "God is subtle, but he is not malicious." So let's scrap Hume's definition of a miracle as "a violation of the laws of nature." The emotionally laden word *violation* prejudices the case. Instead, I propose this definition: *A miracle is a meaningful intervention by God in the laws of nature.*

This definition includes several features that are crucial, I think, to an understanding of miracles.

First, a miracle must come from God, the Cosmic Designer. It must be a deliberate act on the part of the One who wrote the laws of the universe.

Second, a miracle is an intervention, not a violation. When a miracle takes place, it is evidence that God is *involved* in the natural order, not that God is *assaulting* the natural order. A genuine miracle, then, may come as a surprise because it is unexpected—but it will not come as an offense.

Third, a miracle is *meaningful*. It is not random, irrational, or arbitrary; it points us toward a profound truth. It conveys a message from God—usually a message of assurance of God's reality and presence. The best-attested miracles I know are always meaningful, never just for show or sensationalism. I look at the evidence of God's character in the scientific evidence, and I see the essence of rationality and purposefulness. I see a God who conveys a message in the fine-tuned structure of the universe. If that God were ever to intervene in the rational order of the cosmos, I'm sure it would be a *rational* intervention.

There is a scene in the movie *Oh, God!* where God (George Burns) is called to testify in court. When the judge is skeptical of his claim to deity, God says, "What, you want a miracle? I got a cute miracle." He takes out a deck of cards and, with a wave of his hand, the cards disappear. "Happy now?" Point well taken. God does not do cheesy parlor tricks. When God performs a miracle, it is a meaningful and purposeful expression of God's character—not a stunt intended merely to impress.

All it would take to prove that miracles *can* happen is to show that at least one miracle *has* happened. Once you accept the reality of a single miracle, then miracles become possible in principle. And there is *one* miracle that we have *all* experienced and that has been overwhelmingly scientifically verified.

It comes as no surprise, I'm sure, that I'm talking about the universe itself. Of course, some might argue that since the constants of the universe were laid down at the moment of the Big Bang, the Big Bang should be viewed as the *source* of the laws of nature, not an intervention in those laws. Well, that may be true with regard to such cosmic laws as the gravitational force constant or the proton-electron mass ratio. But no scientist would propose that a universe could arise in which, say, $1 + 1 = 3$. Certain fundamental principles of reality must operate in *any* universe.

Take, for example, the Laws of Thermodynamics, which are fundamental principles of reality—as basic and universal as $1 + 1 = 2$. The first two Laws of Thermodynamics are (1) the Law of Conservation of Energy—energy cannot be created or destroyed; and (2) the Law of Entropy—systems tend to evolve toward a state of equilibrium and disorder. Even though the *constants* of the universe might have been structured differently at the instant of the Big Bang, the Laws of Thermodynamics are immutable and invariable. Any physical universe *must* obey these two fundamental principles of reality. And yet—

The Big Bang itself is a glaring contradiction of these laws!

In the first instant of the Big Bang, time and space and energy came into being—a momentary suspension of the first law. At the same instant, the realm of reality (which consisted of no-time, no-space, no-thing, no-order, and no-energy—a realm of absolute entropy and uttermost disorder) suddenly assumed a state of negative entropy and uttermost order. This was a momentary suspension of the second law. From a purely natural

> "*A*ll it would take to prove that miracles can happen is to show that at least one miracle has happened."

point of view, the Big Bang would seem to be a totally uncaused event. But as we saw in an earlier chapter, the anthropic coincidences strongly suggest that the Big Bang was, in fact, an intelligently caused, intelligently engineered event.

The Big Bang was a carefully controlled, delicately balanced explosion that was *purposefully* and *meaningfully* structured in order to bring forth life forms like you and me. We live inside this miracle called the Big Bang, and it continues to blossom all around us in an orderly, rational way. We are all witnesses to Creation.

And there is another miracle that is equally profound and meaningful. It is the miracle of life itself.

The miracle of life

St. Augustine once wrote, "Men go abroad to wonder at the height of mountains, at the huge waves of the sea, at the long courses of the rivers, at the vast compass of the ocean, at the circular motion of the stars; and they pass by themselves without wondering." We seldom stop to consider the fact that *we* are walking miracles, that all of life is a miracle. Our very existence is literally a miracle. In a purely scientific sense, *we should not exist.*

We've all heard of the famous Miller-Urey experiment of 1952. A University of Chicago grad student, Stanley Miller, and his research advisor, Harold Urey, constructed a sealed glass tank filled with methane, ammonia, hydrogen, and water vapor, simulating conditions believed to have existed on the primordial Planet Earth. At regular intervals, an electrical discharge jumped a gap between two electrodes, simulating lightning. Over a week, a yellowish-brown sludge formed in the tank, containing an assortment of compounds, including two of the twenty amino acids used by living cells to form proteins. After the results were announced, the press breathlessly reported that Miller-Urey had created "the building blocks of life."

To this day, high school biology students are taught that Miller-Urey "proves" that the origin of the first living cell was practically inevitable once the first amino acids were formed in the "primordial soup." But as Robert Shapiro, professor of chemistry at New York University and an expert on DNA and genetics, observes in his book *Origins*:

> The very best Miller-Urey chemistry...does not take us very far along the path to a living organism. A mixture of simple chemicals, even one enriched in a few amino acids, no more resembles a bacterium than a small pile of real and nonsense words, each written on an individual scrap of paper, resembles the complete works of Shakespeare.[6]

The problem is that an absolutely astounding number of interlocking systems have to come together at the same instant in just the right way in order for life to arise from nonlife by sheer chance. For example, life requires a cooperative arrangement between proteins and nucleic acids, and there appears to be no way that complex, interlocking systems such as the protein-nucleic acid arrangement can be produced in a single spontaneous step. Physicist Paul Davies, in his book *The Cosmic Blueprint*, observes that unless an incredibly improbable combination of chemicals come together in precisely the right way, it is impossible to spontaneously generate an organism as simple as a virus, which consists of nothing more than a strand of DNA with a protein coat. Davies writes:

> It is possible to perform rough calculations of the probability that the endless breakup and reforming of the [primordial] soup's complex molecules would lead to a small virus after a billion years. Such are the enormous number of different possible chemical combinations that the odds work out at over $10^{2,000,000}$ to one against. This mind-numbing number is more than

the chances against flipping heads on a coin six million times in a row....The spontaneous generation of life by random molecular shuffling is a ludicrously improbable event.[7]

Sir Fred Hoyle and his partner, N. C. Wickramasinghe, once supported the idea of spontaneous generation of life in the Miller-Urey primordial soup of Earth's distant past—then they abruptly changed their minds. Why? Because, like Shapiro and Davies, they did the math and discovered the hopeless improbability of such an occurrence. They found that the odds of randomly assembling all the chemical components in just the right way to make even the most rudimentary living cell would be one in $10^{40,000}$. Hoyle concluded that the likelihood of such a spontaneous event was roughly comparable to the probability that "a tornado sweeping through a junk-yard might assemble a Boeing 747 from the materials therein."[8]

Francis Crick, the Nobel-winning codiscoverer of the molecular structure of DNA, also did the math and concluded that life could not have arisen by chance on the Earth. He wrote a book called *Life Itself*, in which he proposed an idea called *directed panspermia*—the theory that life was seeded on Earth billions of years ago by a spaceship from an advanced civilization. But removing the question of life's origin to another planet does not solve the problem. When the odds of evolving a simple virus by chance are one in $10^{2,000,000}$, there is not enough time in the entire history of the universe, and not enough prebiotic soup on all the planets of the universe, to get the job done.

I'm not suggesting—as the Biblical Creationists do—that the universe was created in six literal twenty-four-hour days back in 4004 B.C. It is a fact that our Earth is four and a half billion years old. It is a fact that life first appeared on the infant Earth about four billion years ago. Yet the evidence strongly suggests that the reality of God is also a fact. Therefore, evolution was most likely the means God used to endow this planet with life—not *blind-chance* evolution, but evolution with a purpose. Life could not have begun, and human beings could not have arisen, by purely random processes.

At this point, a disclaimer is in order. What I am saying here about evolution and the origin of life is not endorsed by leading evolutionist scientists such as Stephen Jay Gould and Richard Dawkins. In fact, it would set their teeth on edge. They would say that I am contaminating pure objective science with subjective religion—and though I would disagree, I do understand why they would think so. To Gould and Dawkins, the suggestion that evolution might be *purposeful* is the rankest heresy.

Stephen Jay Gould has gone to great pains to prevent anyone from thinking that evolution has any purpose whatsoever—least of all the purpose of evolving intelligent beings like ourselves. In his book *Wonderful Life*, he calls human beings "a cosmic accident" and "a wildly improbable evolutionary event," a totally haphazard result of blind, random processes. Gould argues that, even if the evolutionary record could be rewound to the beginning and replayed a million times, it is virtually certain that human life would *not* evolve again. He argues that 99.999 percent of the four-billion-year history of life on this planet took place before the human race even emerged, so how could the purpose of evolution be the appearance of human beings? (As if the time-scales that overwhelm the human mind are at all impressive to the mind of the Cosmic Designer!)

Gould concludes, "No intervening spirit watches lovingly over the affairs of nature....No vital forces propel evolutionary change. And whatever we think of God, his existence is not manifest in the products of nature."[9] And Gould's colleague, Richard Dawkins, opens his book *The Blind Watchmaker* with this statement: "Biology is the study of complicated things that give the appearance of having been designed for a purpose." In another book, *Climbing Mount Improbable*, Dawkins even calls living organisms "designoids." Like Gould, Dawkins is quick to point out that the appearance of design is a *deception*. There is no Cosmic Designer, he says—only the "blind watchmaker" of random mutation and natural selection.

But I have to question that assumption. Since both Gould and Dawkins agree that we clearly find an *appearance* of design and purpose in evolution, isn't it possible that the *reason* evolution appears purposeful is that it *is* purposeful?

After examining the evidence of the anthropic principle, astronomer Fred Hoyle observed, "A commonsense interpretation of the facts suggests that a superintellect has monkeyed with physics, as well as chemistry and biology, and that there are no blind forces worth speaking about in nature."[10] Looking at the evidence of life on Earth, I can only conclude that this same superintellect has monkeyed with evolution as well.

The "Rare Earth" miracle

Just as the universe itself appears to be the result of a series of incredibly unlikely coincidences, so does our own Planet Earth. This is the conclusion that emerges from the book *Rare Earth* by geologist Peter D. Ward and astronomer Donald Brownlee. They convincingly demonstrate that the planet we inhabit is the result of a convergence of highly improbable conditions and events. Some examples:

- Our Earth circles a star on the outskirts of the Milky Way galaxy, just close enough to the galactic core to provide plenty of heavy elements needed for life, but far enough from the galactic core to reduce the chance of collision or orbital disturbance by stars or black holes.

- Our sun is just the right age, size, and type to support life. It formed late enough in the life span of the universe to allow previous generations of stars to cook up heavy elements that make up living beings. The sun's mass is just right to make it sufficiently long-lived for life to evolve, and to create a "habitable zone" of heat and light to support living beings.

- Our Earth is just the right size and has just the right gravity to retain water, while not retaining too much harmful ammonia and methane. It is the right distance from the sun to maintain a stable water cycle. Its orbit is nearly circular, which is important for a stable climate. The tilt of the Earth's axis is just right for moderating global temperatures—a few degrees more or less tilt would result in dangerous temperature extremes. The rotation speed of the Earth is just right to regulate temperatures and winds.

- The Earth's metal core produces a magnetic field that shields land-based life forms from dangerous solar radiation (the dead planet Mars, by contrast, has almost no magnetic field). The Earth's core provides radioactive heat which drives the process of plate tectonics necessary for maintaining life on the planet.

- The Moon's gravity helps regulate the Earth's rotation, which stabilizes climates, making life possible. No other planet in the solar system has a Moon as large (in comparison to the planet) as our own. Other planets (such as Mercury, Venus, and Mars) have no large moons to regulate their rotation, which is partly why those planets are uninhabitable. The Moon was probably formed by a glancing collision with a planet-sized body during the Earth's formative stage. If such lucky collisions are as improbable as scientists believe, then habitable planets like Earth must be extremely rare in the universe.

• Jupiter is the largest planet in our solar system (the mass equivalent of 300 Earths). It is strategically located near the outskirts of our solar system, between the orbits of Mars and Saturn. There, the gigantic gas ball patrols for space debris, sweeping away comets and large asteroids before they can reach Earth and destroy all life. We saw Jupiter perform this lifesaving function in a spectacular way when Comet Shoemaker-Levy crashed into Jupiter in July 1994.

These are just a few of the many factors that make life possible on Planet Earth. Other factors include the nitrogen-oxygen ratio of the atmosphere; the precise levels of CO_2, water vapor, and other greenhouse gases in the atmosphere; the rate of collisions with asteroids and comets; and much more. The "Rare Earth" concept that Ward and Brownlee have demonstrated in their book is like the anthropic principle all over again. It is yet another collection of highly improbable coincidences that converge in a statistically improbable way to create fine-tuned conditions for life to exist. If you tamper with *just one* of these conditions, life on Earth becomes improbable, if not impossible.

So here we have what I call "The Cosmic Hat Trick"—three scientifically attested miracles: the life-giving universe, the life-giving Earth, and life itself. You are a living, breathing miracle, inhabiting a planet that is a miracle of intelligent engineering, wrapped inside a universe that is a miracle of flawless design and purpose. "God never wrought a miracle to convince atheism," wrote Francis Bacon (1551-1626), "because his ordinary works convince it." In reality, the "ordinary works" of the Cosmic Designer are the most spectacular miracles of all. Nature is God's *objet d'art*, God's masterpiece, the tangible expression of the intellect, imagination, and soul of the Cosmic Designer.

Touched by a miracle

Cincinnati Bengals quarterback Jeff Blake fired a pass into the end zone—right into the hands of Green Bay safety LeRoy Butler. With that fourth-quarter interception, the Packers shut down Cincinnati's attempt to come back from a 24 to 10 deficit. A cheer rolled like thunder across Green Bay's Lambeau field—then died to an eerie silence. One Packer was down, writhing in pain.

It was No. 92, Reggie White.

That was December 3, 1995. About three months later, I sat with Reggie in his Knoxville home as he told me what happened that day. As that play began, the Bengals were in a desperate 4th-and-20 situation on the Packers twenty-three-yard line. As the ball was snapped, Reggie came around the corner, beating Bengals tackle Joe Walter off the ball. Walter dove in front of Reggie, trying to cut him at the knees. Reggie leaped to go over Walter, launching himself at Jeff Blake. "I would've had the sack," Reggie told me, "but just when my foot planted, I felt something *pop*."

What popped was Reggie's left hamstring—the tendons behind the hollow of the knee. Those tendons anchor the thigh muscles. "I knew I was hurt bad. The pain wasn't as bad as when I sprung my elbow the year before, but it was bad. I hopped on my right leg a couple times, then went down on the ground. I grabbed the leg and I felt the muscle bunch up in a knot.

"Our head trainer and team doctor came out and looked me over, then LeRoy Butler and Sean Jones helped me off the field. On the sidelines, I thought of guys whose careers were ended by a torn hamstring. I was hoping it was just a bruise or something—but I knew a bruise didn't make a popping sound."

After the game—a lopsided Packer win—the team doctor, Patrick McKenzie, did an MRI and confirmed that the hamstring was torn. Amazingly, Reggie was able to walk on it—but he couldn't play. Dr. McKenzie wanted to schedule Reggie for surgery to reattach the hamstring.

"I'm not gonna have surgery," Reggie replied. "I'm gonna play." He didn't want to be out as the Packers headed into the post-season.

But the doctor knew that No. 92 would not be suiting up the following week in Tampa Bay. Reggie tried out the leg in practice, but he had no strength, no speed. "I felt like Samson with a buzz cut," he told me. Reggie sat out the Tampa Bay game, ending one of the longest iron-man streaks in NFL history—166 games in a row. Worse, with Reggie side-lined, the Packers lost, 13 to 10.

The following week, Reggie yielded to the inevitable. "Okay, Doc," he said. "Guess I need that operation after all."

"Just tell me when," said Dr. McKenzie.

"Make it Sunday," said Reggie. He figured he would just as soon be under anesthesia as sitting on the sidelines in New Orleans.

While he was telling coach Mike Holmgren about the upcoming surgery, Reggie broke down and cried. With the Packers heading into the playoffs, he felt he was letting the team down. "Mike," he said, "I'm sorry."

"There's nothing to be sorry about, Reggie," said Holmgren. "Let's get you fixed up and ready to play next year."

A few days later, one of Reggie's teammates, wide receiver Mark Ingram, told him, "You know, my mom really believes in God. And last night she told me, 'The devil hasn't beaten Reggie White. Something powerful is about to happen.'" Reggie appreciated the encouragement, but he had no faith that anything lay ahead of him but a surgeon's knife.

That night, he was at home in Green Bay, playing with his kids, when he realized that his leg felt surprisingly strong. He flexed it, walked on it, then ran on it. The more he exercised it, the better it felt. He phoned his weight coaches, and they went to the Packers' workout center. He ran sprints and hit the sled, and found he was able to do everything he had done before the injury. The leg continued feeling stronger. "Man," he said, "this is incredible! Let's go tell Mike!"

So Reggie and his weight coaches drove to Coach Holmgren's house. "The way Mike tells it," says Reggie, "it was three in the morning when we got there, but it was really only nine-thirty. I went to the door but before I could knock, the door flung open and there was Mike! I scared him, and he scared me! He didn't know I would be there—he was just coming out to cut the Christmas lights on his house. And I'm like, 'Hey, man! You scared me!' And Mike's like, 'Where'd you come from? Man, I thought you were Santa Claus!' And I said, 'Well, maybe I am, Coach, 'cause I'm ready to play in New Orleans!'

"The next day, I went to the team meeting and sat next to Sean Jones. I was grinning ear to ear. I just couldn't hold it in. And Sean said, 'What?' And I said, 'What *what*?' He said, 'What are you so happy about?' I said, 'I'm just happy 'cause I get to play in New Orleans.' His eyes got *this* big and he said, 'Oh, this is weird, man, this is spooky! I had a dream last night that we were sitting right here and you were telling me this! Are you kidding me, man?' And I said, 'Sean, I'm gonna play.'

"After that, I called a press conference and said that God healed me. Next thing I knew, the TV stations interrupted the soap operas, telling everybody I'd been healed. ESPN ran two video clips back-to-back, first the one where I said, 'I'm not going to play no more this year,' then the one where I said, 'God healed me and I'm gonna play in New Orleans.'

"Some people in the media were skeptical. They said Dr. McKenzie misdiagnosed my leg. Well, I felt insulted on his behalf. Dr. McKenzie didn't make a mistake. When he did that MRI, my leg needed surgery. But now it didn't. So I told the reporters, 'Some of you guys don't believe God healed me. I'm telling you he did. If you've got a problem with that, don't ask me no more questions.'"

Reggie and the Packers went to New Orleans and beat the Saints, 34 to 23. In the stands, a couple of Packer fans held up a sign that read WE BELIEVE. And they weren't just talking about their faith in Reggie White.

I asked Reggie if Mike Holmgren thought it was a miracle. "Oh, he knew it was a miracle, all right," said Reggie. "He told the reporters there was no other explanation for what happened to me."

I then asked Reggie, "With all the problems there are in the world—wars and racial tensions and crime and hunger—why would God take time to heal a football player? Does God care more about you than he cares about all the suffering in the world?"

Reggie thought about that for a few moments, then he said, "All I can say is that God didn't do this for Reggie White. I didn't ask God to heal me—I couldn't believe he would do that. But other people prayed for me to be healed, and God answered so that people's lives would be impacted."

To this day, the hamstring has never been reattached, the muscle is still bunched up in a knot inside his thigh—yet Reggie went on to play three more seasons, including appearances in two Super Bowls. In Super Bowl XXXI, he set a Super Bowl record of three sacks in a single game. A miracle? I'll let you be the judge of that.

Where do miracles come from?

Perhaps you are thinking, "But how does it work? If miracles are real, how does God perform them? And don't tell me, 'He's God, and God can do anything!'" If that is your viewpoint, I agree with you: "God can do anything" is a bad answer. But I believe there is a *good* answer—a logical answer that might account for miracles in a rational, even scientific way.

There was a time, not long ago, when the only realm of nature scientists knew of was the commonsense realm of Newtonian physics. Sir Isaac Newton defined a world of cause and effect, action and reaction, that perfectly matched the experiences and observations we all make on a daily basis. But in 1905, Albert Einstein published his theory of relativity, which completely overturned the old Newtonian realm. In the realm of relativity, the only constant in all frames of reference is the speed of light. Time—a reliable constant in the Newtonian realm—becomes elastic in the Einsteinian realm, passing more slowly for observers in high-gravity regions or observers traveling at near-light speeds.

Soon after, physicists Max Planck, Neils Bohr, and Werner Heisenberg began talking about yet another realm, the realm of quantum mechanics. The quantum realm, like the realm of relativity, also violated the commonsense realm of Newtonian physics. In the quantum world, nothing behaves according to commonsense rules. Quantum particles, like photons and electrons, do not occupy a specific place at a certain time; they are only mathematical probabilities. A particle is not "solid" or "real" in the sense that this book is solid and real; a particle does not move along this or that specific pathway, but along *every* possible pathway at the same time. Each of a pair of twin particles moving in opposite directions seem to "know" when the other is acted upon, even if they are separated by billions of light-years (Einstein called this "spooky action at a distance").

The relativity realm and the quantum realm seem to violate common sense at every turn—yet each has its own mathematical logic and each has proven to be an accurate description of that particular level of reality. Less than a century ago, scientists had no clue that the relativity and quantum realms even existed. Now both are established fact.

I'm convinced that there is another realm of which science is scarcely aware. Like the Einsteinian realm and the quantum realm, this realm has its own logic, and experience has shown it to be real. We know little about it except that it is the realm from which miracles come. A few scientists seem to be groping toward a recognition of its reality. Atheists and skeptics do not recognize this realm, because their mindset filters out all evidence of its existence. Atheism is built upon the *a priori* assumption that no other realm could possibly exist but the one we see, touch, and measure. Astronomer Carl Sagan expressed the atheist view when he wrote, "The cosmos is all that is or ever was or ever will be."[11]

But Sagan was wrong. The cosmos is just *this* level of reality. There is another realm—perhaps *many* other realms, *many* mansions of reality. In *Miracles*, C. S. Lewis pictures reality in just that way. Whereas Carl Sagan sees only one undifferentiated reality ("the cosmos"), Lewis suggests that what we call "nature" or "the cosmos" might be just one floor of a building that houses *many* floors, *many* levels, "Natures piled upon Natures to any height God pleased."[12] Miracles, Lewis goes on to say, are strategic and logical interventions descending from an upper floor to our own floor. God, the Cosmic Designer, does not *invade* our floor of reality; rather, God is *involved* in our floor of reality.

Am I talking about the "supernatural"? No. The skeptic who is rightfully appalled at the thought of the "supernatural"—that irrational fantasy world of ghosts, vampires, and capricious gods—need not be offended by the concept of higher Natures above our own. The Nature where miracles originate is as logical, purposeful, and orderly as our own cosmos. It is, I believe, a Nature that is more profoundly *real* than our own so-called "reality." In fact, I suspect it is so utterly real that the universe we inhabit is the equivalent of a computer simulation by comparison.

After all—what is this thing we call "reality"?

All reality is virtual

Everything we think of as "solid matter" is mostly nothing. Matter is composed of atoms. Atoms are composed of electrons, neutrons, protons, and lots and lots of empty space. What are electrons, neutrons, and protons? They are not hard little objects, like tiny marbles. No, they are probabilities, they are tendencies to exist. They are *partiqles*, not particles. In short, *they are bits of information.*

"Matter is *digital*," observes physicist Stephen L. Gillett, "and it's so because of quantum mechanics."[13] Matter is digital, and so is energy. Even time is thought to be digital, existing as discrete quanta called "chronons." Even our perception of reality is digital. "The human visual system has long been known to be digital," notes physicist Frank Tipler; he adds that for the human mind, "time comes in whole numbers," in discrete digital units, not a continuous flow.[14] Mathematician and computer scientist Roger Penrose observes that the human brain and nervous system operate with "a digital computer-like aspect."[15] The complex structure of a nerve fiber, Penrose explains, is not like an electric wire that carries a continuous current, but like an information gate that transmits digital signals, like the 1s and 0s of a computer.

Scientists have long recognized that the universe, at its most basic level, is made up not of solid "stuff," but of information and mathematical logic. In the 1930s, astronomer-physicist Sir Arthur Eddington said, "The stuff of the world is mind-stuff." Eddington's colleague, Sir James Jeans, put it this way: "The universe appears less and less like a great machine and more and more like a great thought." More recently, physicist John Wheeler (who coined the term "black hole") called *logic* the "nuts and bolts, if you will, out of which the world is made." So reality is made of information, and our minds are designed to process that information in a digital way. In a very real sense, *all* reality is *virtual* reality.

So am I saying that reality is nothing but a vast computer simulation—that the world is nothing but an illusion? No. Let's not trivialize our own existence. The universe is not a computer game, not an illusion. What we call "reality" is not the *ultimate* reality, but it is real enough.

Shankara (A.D. 788–820) was an ascetic Indian philosopher and missionary for Hinduism. He taught that all souls are merely aspects of Brahman, the absolute being who pervades and sustains the universe (roughly equivalent to the western concept of God). Because Brahman is undivided and undifferentiated from human souls, said Shankara, the entire world that we see around us is *maya*, illusion—it has no objective reality.

One day, Shankara and his disciples were walking through the northern city of Varanasi, on their way to bathe in the Ganges River. A few yards in front of them, an elephant suddenly became uncontrollable, broke loose from its handler, and began charging down the narrow street, completely berserk. Shankara and his disciples had to run for their lives to keep from being trampled. Later, a Hindu scholar, an opponent of Shankara's, approached him with a smirk on his face. "O great teacher," said the scholar, "if the world is *maya*, an illusion, as you say, and if the soul is merely an aspect of eternal Brahman, then why did you run? Wasn't the elephant merely an illusion?"

Shankara replied, "Learned friend, the elephant was *maya*, as you say—and so was my running."

A clever riposte—but wrong, in my opinion. The elephant was real. The running was real. *Reality is real*, even though it is made up (like a computer program) of information and logic. I am convinced that the Cosmic Designer interacts with our level of reality much as a computer operator interacts with a computer program. But that doesn't mean our own reality is *maya*. It may not be as real as the *ultimate* reality that lies beyond—but it is real enough. If you are about to be trampled by an elephant, *run!*

As we saw in Chapter 17, many people who undergo a near-death experience report feeling that their out-of-body experience was reality and our own material world was unreal by comparison. Whereas we tend to think of "Heaven" as an insubstantial, unreal place, NDEers who appear to have glimpsed the afterlife say that the here-and-now is what is truly unreal. *Real* reality, they say, is the place where God is, the place to which immortal human souls go after death—and, I submit, the place from which miracles emanate. As real as our own level of reality is, it is like a computer simulation when compared with that even more profound reality that the Cosmic Designer inhabits.

When God intervenes in the operation of our cosmos, it does not mean that the "program" of the universe needs "debugging." A miracle is not a software patch to fix a computer glitch. A miracle is evidence that the Cosmic Designer is operating the program, and that the program is functioning as designed. If a computer operator changes a variable in a spreadsheet program, you don't say that the program is faulty. Computer programs are *designed* to perform operations with variables that can be modified. And so, it would seem, is our universe.

The cosmos is made of digital matter, digital energy, and digital time—a vast array of mathematical variables that can be changed and modified by the One who knows the "source code" of the "program." When the Cosmic Designer alters the variables in the "program" of our universe, it's called a miracle. That is why true miracles are always orderly, meaningful, and purposeful. They always operate according to the rules of logic, even if the Programmer's logic is deeper than our own.

Everyday miracles

Again, once you admit the reality of one miracle (or two or three), you cannot exclude the possibility of other miracles. Obviously, that doesn't mean we should become easy marks for every spoon-bender, faith healer, and snake-oil salesman who comes along. Some so-called "miracles" (such as fire-walking) have perfectly natural explanations. Others are simply con jobs. We owe it to ourselves to be highly skeptical of extraordinary claims. But we shouldn't harden our minds against the possibility of a meaningful intervention in our lives from that other realm of reality.

You might say, "I've never seen a miracle. I doubt I ever will." I have a friend who once said that. I met him over the Internet, and we have been corresponding throughout the entire time I've been writing this book. At one point, early on, I told him that I see miracles almost every day. He posted this response: "You see miracles every day? I've honestly never seen one. Am I not looking hard enough, or are you looking too hard?"

As I considered how to reply, I recalled a quotation by one of my favorite authors, but I couldn't recall the exact wording. I have more than twenty books by this particular author on my shelf, and I didn't have a clue which book it was in. I took down a couple of books, flipped through them, scanning each page, finding nothing. After about twenty minutes of this futility, I prayed aloud, "Help me find that quotation!" Then I took down another book, flipped three or four pages, and *bam*! There it was. For our purposes here, let me paraphrase the quotation as follows: "I believe in God as I believe that the Sun has risen, not only because I see the Sun itself, but because by it I see everything else."

That was my point exactly: Once you become aware of the reality of the Cosmic Designer, you begin to see everything by the light of that awareness. Where once you saw only a world of dead matter, you now see a cosmos alight with consciousness, alive with souls. Where once you only saw randomness, you now see purpose. Where once you only saw coincidence, you now see miracles.

Then it hit me: I had just voiced a prayer for help in finding that quotation—and the quotation had appeared in my hands, *just like that*. Some would call it coincidence. I call it an "everyday miracle"—a minor but meaningful event. It's just the kind of thing the Cosmic Designer would do to say, "Just wanted to let you know I'm here."

So I finished the message to my Internet friend with these words: "You ask, 'Am I not looking hard enough, or are you looking too hard?' Fact is, I don't look hard at all, but I see miracles everywhere. Why?

Because I know the Cosmic Designer is real and involved in my life. It's not just God I see; by the light of God, I see everything else around me. The Sun has risen and by its light I see miracles everywhere."

My Internet friend professed to be an agnostic when that exchange took place. Since then, he has studied the evidence and he now says he believes that the Cosmic Designer is real. He recently told me he now sees miracles, too.

Do miracles really happen? Oh, absolutely. I see them every day.

20

Is Religion Important?

I spent a good portion of my adolescence watching endless reruns of *Star Trek*. My favorites were first-season episodes like "Charlie X" (teenage boy with godlike powers nearly destroys the *Enterprise*) and "The Naked Time" (Mr. Spock breaks down and has a good cry). My favorite episodes all seemed to have one thing in common: a prominent role for Yeoman Janice Rand, played by actress Grace Lee Whitney.

So one of the truly memorable treats of my career was helping Grace Lee Whitney write her memoirs, *The Longest Trek*. I'll never forget the first time I sat down in her home, near Yosemite National Park, while she told me the *real* backstage story of *Star Trek*. I knew that Grace had appeared in only thirteen of the original seventy-two episodes—but until we sat down together and she told me her story, I had never known *why* she left the series.

After a weekend wrap party for the episode "Miri" (in which the *Enterprise* crew discovers a planet of 300-year-old children), Grace was invited to the office of a Desilu executive, ostensibly to talk about expanding her role on the show. Grace and the studio exec were all alone in the E Building at Desilu Studios, and the executive quickly got down to business: If Grace wanted a bigger role on *Star Trek*, all she had to do was have sex with him. She refused—but he wouldn't take no for an answer.

"He locked the door," Grace told me, "and there was nothing I could do. It was late, the building was empty. I could scream, but no one would hear me. He had a dartboard in his office, and he threw darts at me. I thought he was going to kill me. He kept getting angrier and more demanding. Deep down, I knew I was finished on *Star Trek*, but none of that mattered. All I cared about was getting out of that room alive."

Finally, after what seemed like an eternity in hell, the executive got what he wanted. Grace got out alive—but she was destroyed inside.

A few days after the sexual assault, Grace was told that her character had been written out of the show—she was fired from *Star Trek*. Added to the assault on her body and soul was the ruin of her career. Though she managed to get guest-shots on *Mannix* and a few other shows, she found it increasingly hard to get acting jobs after that.

A hole in the soul

Turning to alcohol, drugs, and sex for consolation, Grace began a fifteen-year spiral of bingeing and suicidal depression. She was out of control, and constantly lived with a feeling she described as "holes in my soul with the wind blowing through." By 1981, near the bottom of her downward plunge, Grace found that while she drank more than ever, she couldn't get drunk anymore. The alcohol no longer numbed her pain. Yet, when she tried to stop drinking, she couldn't get sober. "When an alcoholic drinks but can't get drunk," she told me, "or stops drinking but can't get sober, that's the end of the line."

Her health was collapsing. Her gums bled and her hair came out in clumps. She was admitted to a hospital in L.A., suffering from anxiety, hallucinations, delirium tremens, blackouts, and dehydration. "The doctor said my liver was enlarged and distended," Grace told me. "He also found a hole in my esophagus where the gin was eating my flesh away. He said, 'If you don't stop drinking, you'll be dead.' I asked if I had months or years. He said, 'Days.' That really scared me—but I didn't know how to stop drinking."

After her release from the hospital, a friend took her to a Twelve Step recovery meeting in Beverly Hills. "I had been to a couple of meetings before," Grace recalled, "but I hated them. It was like going to church, and I hated church. But *this* meeting was different. This time, I was ready."

The room was full of people she knew—actors, directors, producers. For the first time in her life, she felt she was *home*. She listened as the others told their stories and shared their hope. For the first time in her life, she felt safe and accepted. When she stood and told her story, everyone applauded. "Applause!" she told me, her face beaming. "Just what every actor craves! I felt wave after wave of love wash over me. I wanted what those people had. I wanted to laugh like they laughed. I always thought you needed alcohol to laugh. That night I learned that the music of recovery is laughter."

At the end of the meeting, everyone stood and said the Lord's Prayer together. "I said the prayer," she recalled, "and I suddenly *knew* that God was hearing me. Instantly, my atheist's heart was changed, and my obsession with drinking went away. It was as if I just turned around, and there was God, and I recognized him for the first time. I remember thinking, *Oh, it's you!*"

In her journey of recovery, Grace learned that the only hope for an alcoholic—or for any human being—is a reliance upon a Power greater than ourselves. "I had come to God through a process of elimination," she told me. "I tried everything else first, and God was the last thing on my list, the only thing I hadn't tried. God filled up the holes in my soul."

"There is a God-shaped hole in the heart of everyone," said French mathematician Blaise Pascal, "which cannot be filled by any created thing, but only by God the Creator." That is the same infinitely vast gut-hole that U2's Bono bewails in the song "Mofo": "Looking for to fill that God-shaped hole."

We all have that hole, and we try to stuff it with money or power or fame or drugs or sex or some other thing. It's like trying to fill the ocean with an eyedropper. The Soul that created the universe is infinitely vast, and so is the God-shaped hole within us. If we try to fill an infinite hole with finite stuff, we will always remain empty. Nothing fits and fills that hole but God.

The God module

Where is this "God-shaped hole" located? In 1997, neuroscientists at the University of California at San Diego (UCSD) claimed they had found it in the human brain. The scientists, led by Dr. Vilayanur Ramachandran, studied three groups of volunteers—patients afflicted with temporal lobe epilepsy (TLE), strongly religious people, and nonreligious people. The TLE group had suffered seizures accompanied by intense religious experiences, and also reported being strongly preoccupied with religious thoughts between seizures. UCSD researchers found that the TLE patients appeared to have a malfunction in a particular region of the brain's temporal lobe. They dubbed this region the "God module." It appears that, in non-TLE brains, the God module helps produce belief in God; in people with TLE, the result can be extreme religious obsession and vivid mystical experiences.

The volunteers from all three groups were shown a number of words, including words with sexual, violent, religious, and neutral connotations, and their brain activity was electrically measured. Patients with TLE showed a disproportionately strong reaction to the religious terms. This result led Dr. Ramachandran and his colleagues to conclude that human brains are "hard-wired" for religion in the temporal lobe. Since religious belief is common in all human societies and throughout history, the UCSD researchers speculate that the God module is a Darwinian adaptation to encourage social cooperation and stability, increasing the likelihood of the survival of the human species.

> "The question naturally arises: Did God create the human mind—or did the human mind invent God?"

It's important to underscore, as Dr. Ramachandran and his associates point out, that these are preliminary findings, and much more research needs to be done to verify the existence of the "God module." But assuming that these findings are borne out by further research, the question naturally arises: Did God create the human mind—or did the human mind invent God? When the preliminary results were announced, newspapers reported that scientists had "found the location of God" in the temporal lobe. In other words, God is all in your head.

That would certainly be a reasonable deduction to draw from the evidence if it weren't for one tiny little detail: *The scientific evidence tells us that God exists.* As we have already seen, the anthropic evidence sketches for us an image of an *objectively real* Cosmic Designer who created the cosmos—and human life—with purpose and meaning. Human beings, it appears, were deliberately designed to have a connection with the Cosmic Designer. In light of this evidence, it becomes clear that the God module must have been deliberately installed in us as part of the human blueprint.

The God module creates in us an intrinsic drive for connection with the Infinite. It is just one of a number of modules that are part of the human blueprint. We have a hunger module in our brains; we feel an emptiness inside, and we seek food. We have a sex module in our brains; we feel sexual drives, and we seek sexual expression. We have a God module in our brains; we sense a God-shaped hole in our lives, and we fill it with God—*when the God module functions correctly*.

Of course, just as a person can have an eating disorder or an out-of-control sex drive, the God module, too, can get out of whack. It can cause people to try to fill their God-shaped hole with the wrong things. It can cause people to cling to irrational ideas. It can cause holy wars. It can induce people to give their hard-earned money to hucksters who peddle God on TV. And, paradoxically, an out-of-whack God module can even turn otherwise sensible people into irrational atheists.

I'm not saying all atheists are irrational. Some, quite simply, have never encountered the evidence we've examined in this book. When they are presented with the case for the reality of God, many atheists are persuaded. I've seen it happen.

But there are some atheists who are the unbelieving equivalent of religious fundamentalists. You see it in their eyes—an evangelical zeal for spreading the gospel of unbelief, the Good News of atheism. Everyone needs to believe something; evangelical atheists need to believe in their atheism. Their unbelief is their faith, and they cling to it with a martyr's passion. Perhaps it is their whacked-out God-module that fills them with such zeal and turns them into missionaries of cynicism.

So it would seem that we all have the God module designed into us as part of the human blueprint. I've got a God module. You've got a God module. All God's children got a God module.

Blaming religion

For many people, the word "religion" summons up all sorts of unpleasant images. Religion burned "heretics" at the stake during the Dark Ages (it was corrupt religion, after all, that made the Dark Ages so dark). The medieval Church sold indulgences (which supposedly hosed down the fires of Purgatory) and spent vast sums on ornate cathedrals; the people, meanwhile, lived in squalor. There is the ugly history of the Crusades, the religious pogroms against European Jews, the use of religion to justify human slavery, and the genocidal conquest of the indigenous people of Central and South America.

More recently, religious evil has taken the form of the televangelist sex-and-money scandals of the 1980s; religious cult members dying in mass suicides; religious wars in Northern Ireland, Cyprus, former Yugoslavia, and the Middle East. I'm sure you could add other examples to the list. Fact is, some of the most *evil* people I've ever known have been some of the most *religious* people I've ever known. Religious evil is a fact—but does that mean religion itself is evil?

Let me answer that with an analogy. You could make a good case that Darwin's theory of evolution has enslaved, tortured, and killed more millions than all the religious wars in history. Darwin himself was a racist (the full title of his famous 1859 book was *The Origin of Species by Means of Natural Selection, or, the Preservation of Favored Races in the Struggle for Life*); I find Darwin's opinion of certain races to be unprintable.

Among Darwin's most prominent admirers were Karl Marx and Friedrich Engels. In fact, Marx wanted to dedicate his book, *Das Kapital*, to Darwin, but Darwin declined the honor. Marxism is a profoundly Darwinian belief system, and the Marxist government of the Soviet Union holds the record as the most murderous regime in human history. Lenin's forced collectivism and political purges killed over four million people by 1922; Stalin's forced collectivism and starvation campaign killed more than 8 million Ukrainians. By the time of Stalin's death in 1953, the U.S.S.R. had ruthlessly killed 40 million of its own people.

Add to this the more than thirty-five million Chinese who died under another Marxist, Mao Zedong; the million or more Cambodians who died under Marxist Pol Pot; and the million Ethiopians who were deliberately starved to death in the 1980s under Ethiopia's Marxist regime, and you have a death toll that easily tops seventy-seven million people. Marxism is pure distilled social Darwinism: When the weak are exterminated and the strong survive, that is simply Darwinian natural selection at work.

And there's more. It is no accident that the title of Adolf Hitler's book, *Mein Kampf* (*My Struggle*), echoes the Darwinian struggle for survival.

Darwin's theory of evolution is the philosophical basis for Hitler's racial purity beliefs. Over and over in that book, Hitler talked about *Entwicklung* (evolution), and referred to certain races as "monstrosities halfway between man and ape." With the Darwinist racial view as his rationale, Hitler proceeded to murder twelve million civilians, half of them Jewish. England's great evolutionary scientist, Sir Arthur Keith, was horrified to see a great scientific tool—Darwin's theory of evolution—transformed into a weapon of mass destruction. He wrote that Hitler "consciously sought to make the practice of Germany conform to the theory of evolution."[1] Hitler's Fascist ally, Benito Mussolini, was also a committed Darwinist who believed that war was an evolutionary tool, stimulating human progress by eliminating the weak and inferior.

Add up all the victims of Darwinian social theory and you have a conservative estimate of around ninety million civilian dead. Should we do away with evolution, suppress it, and make sure it is never taught in schools? Should we crucify Darwin as a mass murderer? Of course not. As a scientific theory, evolution has been highly successful and well-verified—just as the reality of the Cosmic Designer has been well-verified. If Darwin, who was a racist, is not responsible for the millions who died under Hitler and Stalin, then the Cosmic Designer is certainly not responsible for the Inquisition or the Crusades.

Atrocities and crimes are simply a function of our human capacity for evil. We cannot blame our bloody history on the teachings of Christ or Moses or Mohammed. Evil people do evil things out of their own cruelty and depravity. Religion doesn't make people torture and kill; fact is, religion teaches forgiveness and love. People do evil because seizing power and inflicting suffering gives them pleasure; religion is merely their pretext. Anyone who blames God or religion for the evil that men do is guilty of shallow thinking.

Do all paths lead to God?

What, then, is religion? I would define religion as a systematic approach to answering the ultimate questions of life. Those questions include:

1. *What is our worldview?* What is the structure of reality?

2. *What is our origin?* Who are we as human beings?

3. *What is our destiny?* Is there anything beyond this life?

4. *What is our purpose?* Is there any meaning to life?

> 5. *What is our authority?* How do we judge right from wrong?

Some would say, "I believe in God, but I don't need a religion. I can go outdoors and commune with nature. I can talk to God wherever I am." Well, maybe so.

But I have found that those who practice an "I-am-a-religion-of-one" approach are often just rationalizing their own spiritual laziness. By contrast, those who are serious about their journey with God tend to focus on that journey in the company of fellow believers. They *want* to be on a path with others who are moving in the same direction. The evidence of the God module shows that we are designed to live in community, not isolation.

But there are so many paths, aren't there? The range of spiritual choices is bewildering. Does it matter which path you follow? Some say, "All paths lead to God." Is that true?

Well, the people who followed Charles Manson thought Charlie was God. Were they on a path to truth? What about the people who followed Jim Jones to their deaths in the jungles of Guyana? Or the people who thought David Koresh was the Second Coming? Or the people of the Heaven's Gate UFO cult? Did those paths lead to God—or to destruction? True, these are extreme examples. But, in a less extreme but equally real way, there are many paths that do not lead to God.

The scientific evidence shows that God is an objective reality. God is not just an idea we can manufacture in our own minds. The religious paths we see around us lead in every which way. They clearly do not all lead toward the same objective reality. So I suggest that the path you choose be selected with care and precision. I am not going to tell you which path you should take—that's not the point of this book. But I will share with you some suggestions for selecting your own path.

1. Seek God with all your might.

Seek God with the same intensity you would pursue any meaningful relationship. If you have problems with God, then by all means argue and debate with God until three in the morning. Scream at God, wrestle with God—but whatever you do, don't let go of God. If there is one truth I have seen verified again and again, it is this: Those who persistently, honestly seek God will find what they are looking for.

2. Seek the truth wherever it leads.

Don't just choose a religion like a child picking an ice cream flavor at Baskin-Robbins. You are finding a path toward objective reality, so seek what *is*, not just what feels good or appeals to you. Build your life on *reality*, not illusion and wishful thinking.

Make sure the path you seek conforms to the evidence. From the evidence, we know that God is not an impersonal force, but a vast and purposeful Soul who is working meaningfully in human lives. So find a worshipping community that seeks connection with the personal God who designed and created the universe, and who answers prayer.

All religions contain *some* truth, but not all religions *are* the truth. Different religions disagree on the nature of God: Is there one God or are there many gods? Is everything God? Are we all gods? Is God personal or is God a cosmic force? Is God involved in our lives, or is God remote and unknowable? As you seek a path of knowing God and connecting with God, the array of religious theories is bound to be confusing. Let me suggest a "reality check" you can apply to various religious systems to see which ones best conform to the verifiable evidence about God:

From the anthropic evidence, we know that God is (in the language of the theologians) *transcendent*. That is, the Cosmic Designer exists apart from and outside of the space-time Creation. In fact, space-time is God's own invention. And from the evidence for the soul, prayer, and miracles, we know that God is also *immanent*. That is, the Cosmic Designer is present and active *within* Creation. God listens when we speak, and God speaks when we listen. So God, who is infinite and incomprehensible in power and scope, is also intimate and knowable as a Person or Soul.

So, based on the evidence, the reality of God is this: God is a *transcendent-immanent, infinite-intimate, incomprehensible-knowable* Being. As you seek a path of knowing God, keep this image of God in your mind. Any path that would lead you away from this understanding of God is a false path. Any path that takes you deeper into this God is a true path.

As John Polkinghorne wrote, "The central religious question is the question of truth. Of course, religion can sustain us in life, or at the approach of death, but it can only do so if it is about the way things really are."[2]

3. Seek a place of worship where people experience God as a daily, practical reality.

Become part of a community of people who are committed to applying spiritual beliefs to everyday life. More than theology, ecstatic emotion, or rote, rite, and ritual, we need to experience the presence and guidance of God in our Monday-through-Friday lives.

But what place of worship should you choose? Large or small, traditional or alternative? Many people find comfort in religious symbols, ceremonies, and rituals. If these things help you to focus on God, then seek a place of worship that employs them.

If you don't find ritual, ceremony, and liturgy to be all that helpful or meaningful, then find a place where God is celebrated in a more relaxed and informal atmosphere. You can experience the reality of God amid candles and stained glass and thousand-year-old hymns, and you can experience God in a rented basement where the "hymns" are played on guitars, drums, and electric bass. If you don't like organized religion, there are plenty of *dis*organized religions to choose from.

The best worship experiences I have known have been in small, close-knit groups that met in homes on weeknights. We discussed our faith together, and applied the concepts and precepts of our faith to our daily struggles. We prayed together and celebrated together. We cared for each other, and supported each other during difficult times. Our small group was a safe place where we could express not only our faith but our doubts.

Some people say that the most real and meaningful worship experiences they've ever had were in Twelve Step recovery groups (such as Alcoholics Anonymous). People who follow the Twelve Steps keep their sobriety by living in moment-by-moment reliance upon what the Steps call "a Power greater than ourselves" and "God as we understood Him." People in Twelve Step groups seem to have recovered what many traditional religions have lost: A daily connection to, and reliance upon, an all-powerful and caring God.

4. Avoid the path of least resistance.

I've often heard people say, "I'm not religious—I'm spiritual." Sounds good—but what does it really mean? Usually the person who says that means, "I don't want to be accountable to God for the way I live my life. I don't want anyone to preach at me and tell me I have to grow and change. I don't want to have to deal with the truth about God or the truth about myself. I want a spirituality that is all warm fuzzies and cosmic vibrations—not hard reality."

I personally have no use for that kind of easy, lazy, so-called "spirituality." *Real* spirituality is about living courageously in a world of hatred and death and injustice. It's about facing the evil and pettiness and selfish impulses that lurk inside each of us, which none of us want to face. It's about *serving God*, not having God serve you.

I can appreciate the feelings of those who say they find God in nature. When I stand on the valley floor at Yosemite National Park, and I see the majesty of El Capitan and Half Dome and Yosemite Falls, I am struck by the awe of what I see. I think, "My God!"—not as the kind of empty expression that so many people use, but as an actual recognition of my connection to the Soul who designed the wonders of this universe.

But an authentic relationship with God doesn't stop with mere feelings of awe and wonder. It doesn't just drink in the beauty of nature or the warm tingly feelings of the soul. Real spirituality looks around at the work that needs to be done, at the sickness and suffering and injustice in the world. An authentic relationship with God puts dirt under your fingernails and an ache in your back. When you truly connect with God, you become God's hands and feet, and through you, God carries out the divine task of feeding and healing and loving people in need. If we claim to be "spiritual," but we've never rolled up our sleeves and done God's work, then what is our "spirituality" really worth?

So beware of the easy path. True spirituality should be hard. God's work is hard work.

5. It's okay to doubt your faith.

It's okay to wonder and agonize and question God. Doubt doesn't make you an unbeliever. Doubt just means you're *thinking*. As Galileo once said, "I do not feel obliged to believe that the same God who has endowed us with sense, reason, and intellect has intended us to forgo their use." Our minds are miniature reflections of God's own immense intellect. I doubt that the Soul who created the cosmos feels threatened by our doubts and questions. The Architect of the human mind would never demand that we sacrifice thinking to believing.

This is not to say that we will ever fully comprehend God. If this great eternal mystery could be fully grasped by the human mind, then God would not be God. A God who is big enough to inspire our faith is big enough to receive our doubts.

One more thing: When you doubt your beliefs, don't forget to doubt your doubts. When a voice comes into your mind, calling into question everything you objectively know about God, ask yourself, "Why did I think that? Is there any objective basis for doubting the objective evidence for God?" Then relax, because doubts are normal—just part of being human. Even atheists have their doubts. At three A.M., in the dark night of the soul, while the sleepless believer asks himself, "What if it's all a lie?" the sleepless atheist asks, "What if it's all *true*?"

6. Build your home around a single faith.

The two most important categories of relationship in your life are (1) your relationship to God and (2) your family relationships. Why would you deliberately choose to set up a clash between those relationships? The person you choose as your life partner should be in sync with the deepest and most sacred part of you—your connection to God. When you and your partner fully and completely share the depths of your faith, it deepens your mutual bond and strengthens the foundation you are building for your life together.

Young people often choose a mate based on attraction alone. *Love will conquer all*, they think. *Besides, God is not that important right now. The only thing that's important is that we love each other.* But a few years pass. Maturity sets in. Children are born. Suddenly, two people who never cared that much about God get *very* religious. Now the holy wars begin: "Hey, don't put the menorah there—you'll set the Christmas tree on fire!"

And what happens to the kids in an interfaith family? Which faith are they raised in? His? Hers? Both? Neither? What holidays do we celebrate? What about pressure and interference from the grandparents? If you impose *both* religions on your children, you inevitably put them in the position of having to choose not between two religions, but between Mom and Dad. The result: Rather than having to choose between Mom's God and Dad's God, they resolve the conflict by becoming atheists or agnostics. Kids reason (justifiably) that your religion wasn't a very important issue when you chose each other, so why should they give it any more consideration than you?

7. In your daily faith experience, relate to God as a person—not as an impersonal force.

Some people would say, "But God isn't a person. I refuse to imagine God as an anthropomorphic stereotype, like an old man in a long white beard." Fine. I'm not suggesting that the Cosmic Designer is a "person" in that sense. But it is clear from the anthropic evidence and the evidence for the soul, prayer, and miracles that the Cosmic Designer is a person in every meaningful sense of the word—a being with specific personality traits, intellect, creativity, and purposefulness.

C. S. Lewis points out that those who deny God's personhood in order to avoid anthropomorphizing God only succeed in substituting some other and equally false notion of God:

> "I don't believe in a personal God," says one, "but I do believe in a great spiritual force." What he has not noticed is that the word "force" has let in all sorts of images about winds and tides and electricity and gravitation....A girl I knew was brought up by "higher thinking" parents to regard God as a perfect "substance"; in later life she realized that this had actually led her to think of Him as something like a vast tapioca pudding. (To make matters worse, she disliked tapioca.) [3]

Our mental conceptions of God tend to be ethereal, incorporeal, and impersonal. The scientific evidence suggests that the exact opposite is true: God is far too definite, too real, too profoundly personal for the vagueness of our language. Everything that is definite, real, and personal about us is really nothing more than an echo of the personhood of God. Our minds are scaled-down versions of the Cosmic Intellect. Our love is a pale glimmering of the Cosmic Love. Our most exalted creations are fumbling imitations of the vast Creation designed by God.

So as you relate to the Soul of the cosmos, don't address your prayers to a force or a substance, but to a Person. How, then, should we picture this Person in our minds?

"I am your father and your mother"

Is it an accident that most of the world's great faiths picture God as a loving, generous father? "You are the children of the Lord your God," says the Hebrew Torah (Deuteronomy 14:1). And the founder of the Christian faith not only told us the story of "The Prodigal Son and the Loving Father," but also taught us to pray, "Our Father in heaven, hallowed be Your name..." The name Jesus used when praying to God was "Abba," an Aramaic term meaning "Daddy" or (more childlike still) "Da-Da."

The image of God's fatherhood dovetails with our emotional and spiritual need as human souls. For those, like me, who were raised by a good and loving father, the image of God as father creates an instant association of a guide, mentor, teacher, provider, example, encourager, and friend. For those whose earthly father was absent, neglectful, or abusive, knowing God as father allows you to have a second chance at being parented by a loving father.

My friend Grace Lee Whitney (whose story opened this chapter) spent most of her lifetime thinking she had no mother or father. When Grace was seven, her mother took her into her lap and said, "Grace, when you were a baby, we chose you. I didn't give birth to you. Another woman was your real mother, but she couldn't keep you, so we adopted you."

As Grace told me this story, she said, "I looked at my mother in shock! She tried to make adoption sound like a good thing, and it is—but I didn't understand. To me, it was as if the bottom had dropped out of my world. I said, 'You mean you're *not* my mother?' And my mother said, 'No, I'm not.'"

"Then," asked seven-year-old Grace, "who are you?"

"I'm your *adopted* mother."

"Where is my *real* mother? And where is my *real* father?"

"I don't know."

"Just like that," Grace told me, with a snap of her fingers, "my safe little world was gone. Suddenly, I didn't know who I was or where I belonged. I felt all alone in the world. I thought there must have been something terribly wrong with me for my birth mother to give me away."

Grace's mother had tried to tell her about the adoption in a gentle and loving way. But adults forget that children put their own spin on what they hear. "Every positive word my mother told me," Grace recalls, "I rewrote as a negative. Around that time, I also figured out there is no Santa Claus. Well, I'd already learned that my own identity was a myth and that Santa Claus was a lie. What's next? Then it hit me that everything I'd learned in Sunday School must be a lie, too. That's when I stopped believing in God."

She remained an atheist for most of her life, during her career as an actress in films like *Some Like It Hot* and *Irma La Douce*, during her tour of duty aboard the Starship *Enterprise*, during her descent into the deepest hell of alcoholism and sex addiction, and right up until the moment she walked into a Twelve Step recovery meeting in Beverly Hills. In that meeting, when she said the prayer that begins, "Our Father in heaven, hallowed be Your name..."*that* was the moment she *knew* God was there. Instantly, her angry atheist's heart was transformed.

Grace had found God—but it would take time for her to fully grasp the fact that God was truly her *Father*. A little more than two years into her recovery, Grace's mother lay dying in a Los Angeles hospital. This was the same woman who had sat her down at age seven and told her, "I'm your *adopted* mother."

"I knew she was dying," Grace told me. "I went to visit her at the hospital. She was delirious. As I stood by her bed, she began talking to me as if I were a little girl. And it was so strange, because I actually began to *feel* like a little girl again. I felt I was shrinking down into the body of a small child, and I was looking at her through a child's eyes."

And there, at her mother's deathbed, the whole dialogue came back to her from the mists of her childhood: "You mean, you're *not* my mother?" "No, I'm not." "Then who are you?" "I'm your *adopted* mother." "Where is my *real* mother? And my *real* father?" "I don't know."

After this conversation replayed in her mind, Grace said aloud, "Well, if you're not my mother, then who am I?" The dying woman in the hospital bed did not answer.

That afternoon, Grace went to a recovery meeting and told the group that for the past fifty years, she had not known who she was, where she came from, or where she belonged. "I started to cry," Grace told me. "Everybody wanted to reach out to me and be my family, but there was something missing inside me that even the group could not supply."

The next morning, she got up to go to work. "I got in my car and started out for the office," she recalls. "As I drove across Laurel Canyon, the pain grew worse by the moment. It was the pain of feeling abandoned by my birth mother. I was crying so hard, I couldn't see the road. The pain doubled me up, like a knife in my middle. I pulled off the road and screamed, 'If she's not my mother, then who am I?!'"

And then Grace heard a voice.

"It seemed to come from outside the car," she recalled. "I knew that voice. It said, 'I am your father and your mother, and I will never leave you or abandon you.' The moment I heard that voice, I felt a sense of peace wash over me. And ever since then, I have known who I am and where I belong."

I have never heard God speak in an audible voice. Most of us never will. But for all of us, there is a still, small voice that whispers to us. It tells us who we are and where we belong—if we are listening.

If we follow that voice and go where it leads us, we will one day understand the meaning of this journey called Life. When we do, every mystery will be solved, all our wondering will be at an end—

And our souls will be truly satisfied at last.

Notes

Chapter 1: *Does Character Really Matter?*
   1. Lyall Watson, *Dark Nature: A Natural History of Evil* (New York: HarperCollins Publishers, 1995), p. 287.
   2. Mark Clayton, "A Whole Lot of Cheatin' Going On," *The Christian Science Monitor*, 19 January 1999, p. 17.
   3. Benjamin Kleinmuntz, "True Lies: The Dishonesty of Honesty Tests," *The Humanist*, 17 July 1995, pp. 4ff.
   4. Rebecca Trounson, "King Hussein was Jordanians' Beloved Benefactor, The Star (of Jordan), 11 February 1999; Howard Schneider, "A New King Shows His Will," *The Washington Post*, 12 May 1999, p. A21; Marilyn Gardner, "Walking a Mile in Another's Shoes," *The Christian Science Monitor*, 2 February 2000, p 16.
   5. Loren Lomasky, "Generosity: Virtue in Civil Society (book review)," *Reason*, 1 May 1998, p. 58.

Chapter 2: *How Do I Become Successful?*
   1. Thomas J. Stanley and William D. Danko, *The Millionaire Next Door* (New York: Pocket Books, 1996), pp. 1-2.
   2. Stanley and Danko, pp. 59-60.
   3. Cited by Eric Black in "Debating the wage gap," *Minneapolis Star Tribune*, 22 June 1996, pp. 12A.

Chapter 3: *How Can I Increase My Luck?*
   1. Max Gunther, *The Luck Factor* (New York: Macmillan, 1977), p. 25.
   2. Joe Kita, "Beat the odds," *Men's Health*, 1 April 1995, pp. 102-108.

Chapter 5: *How Can I Learn to Stop Worrying?*
   1. Gavin De Becker, "What Americans Are Afraid of Today," *USA Weekend*, 24 August 1997, p. 4; the USA Weekend poll of 1,009 adults was conducted in June 1997 by Opinion Research Corporation International; margin of error: ± 3 percentage points; job-related items reflect the responses of 665 adults who work outside the home.
   2. Survey cited by Eleanor Bailey, "Doctor, I'm Dying Again," *Independent on Sunday*, 16 June 1996, p. 6.
   3. Pamela Warrick, "Do Worry, Be Happy: The Benefits of Worrying," *Redbook*, 1 March 1994, p. 70.
   4. Jamie Talan, "Worry: Learning How to Control It, Rather Than Letting It Control You," *Newsday*, 24 November 1997, p. B13.

Chapter 6: *What is Love?*
   1. C.S. Lewis, *The Four Loves*, collected in *The Inspirational Writings of C.S. Lewis*, New York: Inspirational Press, 1991, p. 249.
   2. Richard Selzer, *Mortal Lessons: Notes in the Art of Surgery* (New York: Simon & Schuster, 1976), pp. 45-46.

Chapter 7: *How Can I Build a Better Relationship?*
   1. Harville Hendrix, *Getting the Love You Want* (New York: HarperCollins, 1990), p. 35.
   2. Hendrix, p. 39.
   3. M. Scott Peck, *Denial of the Soul* (New York: Harmony Books, 1997), p. 178.

Chapter 8: How Can I Get Past Feeling Angry?

1. Carol M. Ostrom and Lee Moriwaki, "Anger is All the Rage: At Home, At Work, On the Road, We Are Collectively Losing It," *St. Louis Post-Dispatch*, 9 May 1995, p. 1D.

2. Derrick Henry, "Health Watch: Hotheads Likely to be Male, Experts Say," *The Atlanta Journal and Constitution*, 26 March 1998, p. E3; Carol M. Ostrom and Lee Moriwaki, "Anger is All the Rage: At Home, At Work, On the Road, We Are Collectively Losing It," *St. Louis Post-Dispatch*, 9 May 1995, p. 1D.

3. Charlotte Latvala, "V is for (Very) Volatile," *Cosmopolitan*, 1 November 1996, p. 220.

4. Christopher Scanlon, "Daddy's Rage," *The Fresno Bee*, 31 October 1999, pp. G1,G3.

Chapter 9: Do I Have to Forgive Others?

1. Compiled from reports in the following sources: Leonard Pitts / Miami Herald, "Sometimes You Know That It Really Is the Voice of God," *The Dallas Morning News*, 29 September 1996, p. 7J; Associated Press, "Man Who Survived Abduction is Kidnapper's Only Friend at Death," *The Dallas Morning News*, 6 October 1996, p. 11A; Associated Press, "Victim Befriends Elderly Man Who Kidnapped Him," electronically retrieved at http://www.standardtimes.com/daily/09-96/09-13-96/a08wn045.htm; Rick Brunson, "Victim, Kidnapper Pray Together 20 Years After Brutal Crime," electronically retrieved at http://www.newmanmag.com/stories/na197112.htm.

2. Jonathan Dube, "Forgiving Columbine: Should We Forgive Eric Harris and Dylan Klebold?," ABC News, 20 April, 1999, electronically retrieved at http://www.abcnews.go.com/sections/us/DailyNews/columbine_forgiveness000420.html.

3. Alicia Brooks Waltman, "Everett Worthington, Jr.—In His Own Words: Healing Power," *People*, 14 June 1999, p. 93.

Chapter 10: How Can I Forgive Myself?

1. Dru Scott, Ph.D., *How to Put More Time in Your Life* (New York: Signet, 1980), p. 35.

Chapter 11: How Can I Find Happiness?

1. Viktor Frankl, *Man's Search for Meaning: An Introduction to Logotherapy*, 4th ed. (Boston: Beacon Press, 1992), p. 140.

2. Statistics cited in "Science, Medicine and Uncritical Scribes," *The Toronto Star*, 16 January 1999.

Chapter 12: What Is Truth?

1. Kathy Myatt, R.N., M.S.N., "Truth," electronically retrieved at http://www.dtl.org/dtl/article/truth.htm.

2. John Leo, "A No-Fault Holocaust," *U.S. News & World Report*, 21 July, 1997, p. 14.

3. Thomas Lickona, "The Decline and Fall of American Civilization," *The World & I*, 1 June 1996, p. 284.

4. Kenan Malik, "Scourge of the Postmodernists," *New Statesman*, 19 June 1998, pp. 21ff.; Dinshaw K. Dadachanji, "The Cultural Challenge to Scientific Knowledge," *The World & I*, 1 January 1998, p. 172; "You Can't Follow the Science Wars Without a Battle Map," *The Economist*, 13 December 1997.

5. Kenan Malik, "Scourge of the Postmodernists," *New Statesman*, 19 June 1998, p. 22.

6. Harvey Mackay, United Feature Syndicate, "Truth is Still the Best Way to Improve Your Business," *The Arizona Republic*, 11 April 1999, p. D6.

Chapter 13: What Is the Meaning of Life?

1. Viktor Frankl, *Man's Search for Meaning: An Introduction to Logotherapy*, 4th ed. (Boston: Beacon Press, 1992), pp. 109-110.

2. Frankl, p. 85, emphasis in the original.

3. Frankl, p. 144.

Chapter 14: *Why Is There Evil in the World?*
1. Kristine Vick, "Return to Columbine," electronically retrieved at http://www.cbn.org/newsstand/cwn/990812e.asp.
2. C. S. Lewis, *A Grief Observed* (New York: Bantam Books, 1980), p. 5.
3. Viktor Frankl, *Man's Search for Meaning: An Introduction to Logotherapy*, 4th ed. (Boston: Beacon Press, 1992), p. 122.
4. From the 1981 motion picture *Time Bandits* (Director: Terry Gilliam; Writers: Michael Palin, Terry Gilliam).
5. Martin L. Bard, "The Impossibility of Deity," *The American Atheist*, Volume 37, No. 1, Winter 1998-1999, electronically retrieved at http://www.americanatheist.org/win98-99/T2/bard.html.
6. M. Scott Peck, *People of the Lie: The Hope for Healing Human Evil* (New York: Simon & Schuster, 1983), p. 244.
7. Peck, *People of the Lie*, p. 205.
8. M. Scott Peck, *Denial of the Soul* (New York: Harmony Books, 1997), p. 151-152.

Chapter 15: *How Can I Get Past My Fear of Death?*
1. Rabbi Ben Kamin, *The Path of the Soul: Making Peace With Mortality* (New York: Penguin/Plume, 1999), p. 26.
2. Kamin, *The Path of the Soul*, p. 13.
3. Michael P. Kube-McDowell, reply to Brian Marasca, CompuServe Science Fiction & Fantasy Forum, 31 May 1991.
4. Frank R. Zindler, "The Prospects For Physical Immortality," *The American Atheist*, Volume 37, No. 1, Winter 1998-1999, electronically retrieved at http://www.americanatheist.org/win98-99/T2/zindler.html.
5. Ibid.
6. Don Lattin / *San Francisco Chronicle*, "Raging Against the Dying of the Light: Attitudes Toward Death That She Espoused Provide Psychiatrist Little Comfort," *The Dallas Morning News*, 6 June 1997, p. 1C.
7. Cathy Hainer, "Living Fully is Kübler-Ross' Best Advice," *USA Today*, 11 August 1997, p. 6D.
8. Maureen West, "Expert on Dying Finds Life: Elisabeth Kübler-Ross Rallies During Recovery from 6th Stroke," *The Arizona Republic*, 9 August 1998, p. E1.

Chapter 16: *Does God Exist?*
1. David Alexander, "Gene Roddenberry: Writer, Producer, Philosopher, Humanist," *The Humanist*, March/April 1991, Vol. 51, No. 2, p. 6.
2. George Greenstein, *The Symbiotic Universe* (New York: Morrow, 1988), p. 25.
3. Richard D. Meisner, "Universe—the Ultimate Artifact?," *Analog Science Fiction/Science Fact*, Vol. 107, No. 4, April 1987, pp. 63-64.
4. Michael D. Lemonick, "Echoes of the Big Bang," *Time*, 4 May, 1992, p. 62.
5. Paul Davies, *God and the New Physics* (New York: Simon & Schuster, 1983), pp. 179,181.
6. Roger Penrose, *The Emperor's New Mind* (New York: Oxford University Press, 1989), p. 326, emphasis in the original.
7. Greenstein, p. 41.
8. Meisner, p. 64.
9. Meisner, p. 59.
10. Meisner, p. 60.
11. Greenstein, pp. 43-44.
12. Greenstein, p. 89.
13. Greenstein, p. 27.
14. Greenstein, p. 87.
15. Greenstein, p. 197.
16. Alexander, p. 8.

Chapter 17: What Is the Soul?

1. M. Scott Peck, *Denial of the Soul* (New York: Harmony Books, 1997), p. 133.

2. Isaac Asimov, "The Subtlest Difference," *Science and the Paranormal*, ed. George O. Abell and Barry Singer (New York: Scribner, 1981), p. 158.

3. George Greenstein, *The Symbiotic Universe* (New York: Morrow, 1988), p. 216.

4. Paul Davies, *God and the New Physics* (New York: Simon & Schuster, 1983), p. 173.

5. Paul Davies, *The Mind of God: The Scientific Basis for a Rational World* (New York: Simon & Schuster, 1992), pp. 158-159.

6. Greenstein, pp. 223, 230, emphasis in the original.

7. Isaac Asimov, *Quasar, Quasar, Burning Bright* (NY: Doubleday, 1978), pp. 231-233.

8. Peck, p. 187.

9. Ian Wilson, *The After Death Experience* (New York: Morrow, 1987), pp. 117,121.

10. Brendan I. Koerner; Joshua Rich, "Is there life after death?," *U.S. News & World Report*, 31 March 1997, p. 58.

11. Kenneth Ring, *Life at Death: A Scientific Investigation of the Near-Death Experience* (New York: Coward, McCann, and Geoghegan, 1980), p. 210.

12. Carl Sagan, *Broca's Brain: Reflections on the Romance of Science* (New York: Random House), pp. 305-306.

13. Elisabeth Kübler-Ross, *On Children and Death* (New York: Touchstone, 1997), p. 210.

14. Kübler-Ross, ibid.

15. Kübler-Ross, pp. 210-211.

16. Kübler-Ross, p. 220.

Chapter 18: Does Prayer Really Work?

1. Randolph C. Byrd, M.D., "Positive Therapeutic Effects of Intercessory Prayer in a Coronary Care Unit Population, *Southern Medical Journal*, July 1988 (Vol. 81, No. 7), p. 829.

2. Harris, W.S., et al, "A Randomized, Controlled Trial of the Effects of Remote, Intercessory Prayer on Outcomes in Patients Admitted to the Coronary Care Unit," The *Archives of Internal Medicine*, Vol. 159, No. 19, 25 October 1999, pp. 2273-2278, electronically retrieved at http://archinte.ama-assn.org/issues/v159n19/full/ioi90043.html.

3. Eric Adler, Knight Ridder, Athens Newspapers, Inc., "Heart Patients May Benefit From Other People's Prayers," electronically retrieved at http://www.onlineathens.com/stories/102799/hea_1027990042.html.

4. Harris, et al.

Chapter 19: Do Miracles Really Happen?

1. Sean O'Neill, "Inquiry Into Recruits' Baptism of Fire," *The Daily Telegraph* (London), 15 July 1998.

2. National Public Radio's "Weekend Saturday," 4 July 1998.

3. David Hume, *An Enquiry Concerning Human Understanding*, L. A. Selby Bigge, ed. (Oxford: Clarendon Press, 1902), p. 114.

4. Stephen King, *It* (New York: Viking Press, 1986), p. 430.

5. C.S. Lewis, *Miracles*, collected in *The Best of C.S. Lewis*, Washington, D.C.: Canon Press, 1974, p. 293.

6. Robert Shapiro, *Origins: A Skeptic's Guide to the Creation of Life on Earth* (New York: Summit, 1986), p. 116.

7. Paul Davies, *The Cosmic Blueprint* (New York: Simon & Schuster, 1988), p. 118.

8. Quoted in Shapiro, p. 127.

9. Stephen Jay Gould, "In Praise of Charles Darwin," from *Darwin's Legacy*, Charles L. Hamrum, ed. (San Francisco: Harper & Row, 1983), pp. 6-7.

10. Quoted by Richard D. Meisner, "Universe—the Ultimate Artifact?," *Analog Science Fiction/Science Fact*, Vol. 107, No. 4, April 1987, p. 63.

11. Carl Sagan, *Cosmos* (New York: Random House, 1977, p. 4.

12. Lewis, *Miracles*, p. 352.

13. Stephen L. Gillett, Ph.D., "Digital Matter," *Analog*, February 1999, p. 37.

14. Frank J. Tipler, *The Physics of Immortality* (New York: Anchor Books, 1994), p. 32.

15. Roger Penrose, *The Emperor's New Mind* (New York: Oxford University Press, 1989), p. 392.

Chapter 20: Is It Important to Have a Religion?

1. Sir Arthur Keith, *Evolution and Ethics* (New York: G.P. Putnam's Sons, 1947), p. 230.

2. John Polkinghorne, *Quarks, Chaos, and Christianity* (New York: Crossroad, 1996), p. 97.

3. C.S. Lewis, *Miracles*, collected in *The Best of C.S. Lewis*, Washington, D.C.: Canon Press, 1974, p. 272.

In Appreciation...

What a journey this has been!

The long process of writing this book has not only involved my family and many long-standing friends, but it has also brought me many new friends. So I want to gratefully acknowledge all of those who have left their mark upon these pages.

First, thanks to my wife, Debbie, and my children, Bethany and Ryan, who continually encourage me, teach me, and tolerate my assorted manias. From my family, I draw the energy to start each writing day with confidence and enthusiasm. They keep me going, they keep me young.

I will always be grateful to my parents, Lee and Twyla Denney, for endowing me with the gifts of optimism, perseverance, and the love of knowledge and wisdom. Their influence is like an invisible watermark on these pages—it can only be seen when held up to the light.

I especially appreciate my publisher, Stephen Blake Mettee, for believing in this idea and for giving me the benefit of his wisdom and insight in shaping these chapters (Steve, I honestly wouldn't have entrusted this book to anyone but you). Also, thanks to David Marion, senior editor at Quill Driver Books, for his perceptive advice and untiring efforts on behalf of this book.

I have drawn inspiration and encouragement from my friend of thirty years, Fred Judkins. He makes me laugh; he makes me *believe*. He never ceases to astonish me, and his life challenges me to keep venturing out to the far reaches and outer edges of my convictions.

I'm grateful to Kimberly Clark Sharp, author of *After the Light*, for giving generously of her time and her story, so that I could better understand this deep mystery called the Near Death Experience.

I'm profoundly indebted to the many people I have conversed with over the years—friends who have enlarged my understanding of the issues in this book: Super Bowl champions Reggie White and Bob Griese; Denver Broncos quarterback Brian Griese; supermodel Kim Alexis; actress Grace Lee Whitney; the Exalted Mystic Mage of the Orlando Magic, Pat Williams; recording artist Barry McGuire; super-CEO Gregory Slayton (of ClickAction); my "Doctor of Enthusiasm," Bert Decker (of Decker Communications, Inc. and Bold Assurance); my "Doctor of Motivation," Dru Scott Decker (of Dru Scott Associates); various "Doctors of the Soul," psychologists, psychiatrists, counselors, and clergy, including James Osterhaus, Leighton Ford, Phil Brewer, Brian Newman, Kenneth F. Parker, Steve Williams, and my longtime friend and encourager Joe Pettit.

The ideas in this book have been fine-tuned through literally hundreds of conversations I've had, either face-to-face, or by phone, or over this global miracle called the Internet. Brian Gates and Wade Williams, Jr., not only engaged these ideas in endless hours of conversation, but also read and critiqued the manuscript.

Many others have helped me test-drive the concepts in this book through frank give-and-take on various Internet forums. They include: Conor Northup, Jim Coomber, Brian Flynn, and a number of anonymous souls scattered around the globe—people known to me by such names as Paradoctor, DrWho, AstroSkeptic, The Mirrorball Man, LizardLaugh, Kurgan, Ikhnaton, TrinitY2K, Cracou, Waynehead, Q2, Mr Light, Floydjoy, Captain Kash, Plm135, Ensign Red Shirt, Tw@in, King of Borg, Opinionated Trekkie, Admiral, The Lone Ensign, Core, Khiran, BlueAloe, Maxi, Tusock, Blueberrie, Susannah, Sha-ka-ree, Aeolian, Barcode, Necromancer, TheEmissary, Scourge, Lord Coal, chewie's hairbrush, Watto T, BeastMaster, Khamier, Argath, Tyrael99, Jat'Kidal, Raen, ShadeShifter, Jericho, Jedi Calypso, Binks, and Arcturis Apt Pendragon.

This is not meant to suggest that all the people named (or pseudo-named) above would necessarily agree with all of the ideas in this book. A few of them contributed by contending *against* my ideas—and for their help in testing these ideas under fire, I am grateful. Also, if there are errors or oversights in these pages, the fault is entirely mine.

Finally, my thanks to you, the reader, for purchasing and spending some of your valuable time with *Answers to Satisfy the Soul*. Writing this book has changed my life. I hope that reading it has provided you with some pleasure and some measure of reward. I hope you have experienced a bit of the same electric tingle I felt when I first discovered the truth described by Orson Scott Card in *Speaker for the Dead*:

"How suddenly we find the flesh of God within us after all, when we thought we were only made of dust."

—Jim Denney

About the Author

Jim Denney is a freelance writer with more than 45 published books to his credit. He has collaborated with numerous authorities and celebrities from many fields, including sports, entertainment, business, psychology, and religion.

He worked with Super Bowl champion Reggie White on the football star's autobiography, *In the Trenches*, and with Orlando Magic executive vice president Pat Williams on his motivational classic *Go For the Magic* (each sold over 100,000 copies in hardcover). Another book Denney wrote with Pat Williams, *The Magic of Teamwork*, garnered praise from such notables as novelist James A. Michener ("a wise and needed book"), L.A. Lakers head coach Phil Jackson ("an outline for success in any business"), and CNN's Larry King ("a classic, one-of-a-kind...four stars!").

Jim Denney has also worked with supermodel Kim Alexis on her book *A Model for a Better Future* and with Star Trek actress Grace Lee Whitney on her Hollywood memoir *The Longest Trek*.

He and his family enjoy living in California amid natural scenic wonders, endless sunshine, earthquakes, and rolling blackouts.

Would you like to learn more about the answers in this book? Would you like to meet the author? Ask him questions? Argue with him? Jim Denney is just a click away. Visit him at:

WWW.*denneybooks*.com